A Medicinal Herb Guide

Healthy Digestion

A Natural Approach to Relieving Indigestion, Gas, Heartburn, Constipation, Colitis, and More

David Hoffmann, E

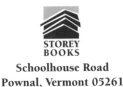
STOREY
BOOKS
Schoolhouse Road
Pownal, Vermont 05261

The mission of Storey Communications is to serve our customers
by publishing practical information that encourages
personal independence in harmony with the environment.

This publication is intended to provide educational information for the reader on the covered subject. It is not intended to take the place of personalized medical counseling, diagnosis, and treatment from a trained health professional.

Edited by Deborah Balmuth and Robin Catalano
Cover design by Meredith Maker
Cover art production and text design by Betty Kodela
Text production by Jennifer Jepson Smith
Illustrations by on pages 2, 19, 26, 30, 35, 50, 65, 81, 85, 93, 95 (bottom), and 102 by Sarah Brill; pages 21, 23, 29, 43, 52, 56, 58, 62, 71, 74, 84 (bottom), 87 (top), 90, 95 (top), 96, 100, 101, 104, 106, and 107 (bottom), by Beverly Duncan; page 24 by Brigita Furhmann; page 77 by Alison Kolesar; page 83 by Charles Joslin; pages 84 (top), 86 (bottom), 91, and 103 by Mallory Lake; page 85 (bottom) by Myla Scudder; page 87 (bottom) by Douglas Paisley; page 107 (top) by Regina Hughes; pages 111, 113, and 114 by Randy Mosher; page 92 by LaVonne Francis.
Indexed by Susan Olason, Indexes & Knowledge Maps

Printed in the United States by Versa Press
10 9 8 7 6 5 4 3 2 1

Library of Congress Cataloging-in-Publication Data

Hoffmann, David, 1951–
    Healthy digestion: a natural approach to relieving indigestion, gas, heartburn, constipation, colitis, and more / David Hoffmann
        p.   cm. — (Storey medicinal herb guide)
    Includes bibliographical references and index.
        ISBN 1-58017-250-4 (pbk. : alk. paper)
        1. Indigestion—alternative treatment. 2. Digestive organs—Diseases—Alternative treatment. 3. Herbs—Therapeutic use. I. Title. II. Medicinal herb guide
RC827.H64 2000
616.3'06—dc21   99-089106
                                                                                            CIP

CONTENTS

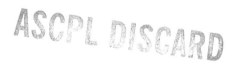

DEDICATION

Thank you Lolo — you know why!

This book is also dedicated to all my brothers and sisters who grew up experiencing the dubious joys of English cooking. Yes, there is life beyond the "chip butty"...

UNDERSTANDING THE DIGESTIVE SYSTEM

Herbal medicine is uniquely suited for the treatment of illness of the digestive system. Throughout the natural world food is medicine, and the same concept applies to herbs — the ultimate medicinal food.

Much of the digestive system illness in our society is simply due to abuse. Today's average Western diet includes a preponderance of overly processed foods, a high proportion of chemical additives, and the direct chemical irritation of alcohol, carbonated drinks, and tobacco. In this context it is easy to see why herbal remedies are so helpful in healing digestive problems; the soothing of demulcents, healing of astringents, and general toning of bitters do much to reverse the damage we do every day.

WHAT IS THE DIGESTIVE SYSTEM?

The digestive system is a series of hollow organs joined in a long, twisting tube — known as the alimentary canal — from the mouth to the anus. Inside the tube is a lining called the mucosa, which in the mouth, stomach, and small intestine contains glands that produce digestive juices. The liver and the pancreas are also part of the system, producing juices that reach the intestine through small tubes.

The Process of Digestion

The food we eat is not in a form that the body can use as nourishment. It must be broken down into smaller molecules of nutrients that the blood can absorb and carry to the cells of the body. Digestion breaks down food and drink into their smallest parts so that the body can use them to build and nourish cells and to provide energy. The process, which begins in the mouth with chewing and swallowing and is completed in the small intestine, involves the mixing of food, its movement through the digestive tract, and the chemical breakdown of its large molecules into

The Digestive System

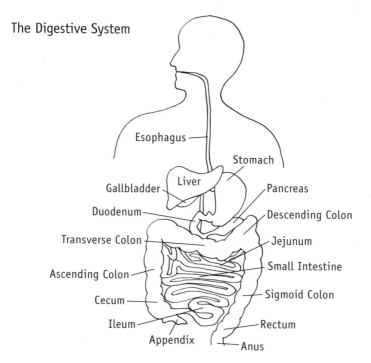

Esophagus
Stomach
Gallbladder
Liver
Pancreas
Duodenum
Descending Colon
Transverse Colon
Jejunum
Ascending Colon
Small Intestine
Cecum
Sigmoid Colon
Ileum
Rectum
Appendix
Anus

smaller molecules The chemical process varies somewhat for different kinds of food.

The digestive system's hollow organs contain muscles that enable their walls to move. This involuntary movement, called peristalsis, not only forces the contents forward but also mixes them. When we swallow, peristalsis begins. The muscles then contract and narrow, propelling the food particles and fluid down the length of the alimentary canal in slow waves.

The esophagus connects the throat above with the stomach below. At the junction of the esophagus and stomach, a ringlike valve closes the passage between the two organs. As the food travels down the esophagus and approaches the closed ring, the surrounding muscles relax and allow the food to pass through.

The food then enters the stomach, which performs several functions. The stomach stores the swallowed food and liquid and produces digestive juices. Muscle action in the lower part of the stomach mixes the contents of the stomach. Finally, the stomach slowly empties its contents into the small intestine. Several factors affect this emptying, including the nature of the food and the degree of muscle action of the emptying stomach and the small intestine. As the food is digested in the small intestine and dissolved by the juices from the pancreas, liver, and intestine, muscle action continues to mix the contents of the intestine and push them forward.

Finally, all of the digested nutrients are absorbed through the intestinal walls. The waste products of this process include undigested parts of the food, known as fiber, and older cells that have been shed from the mucosa. These materials are propelled into the colon, where they remain, usually for a day or two, until they are expelled as feces through a bowel movement.

The production of digestive juices is a vital function of the digestive system. The salivary glands in the mouth start that process. An enzyme in saliva begins to digest the starch in food into smaller molecules. The next set of glands involved in digestion is in the lining of the stomach. These gastric glands produce stomach acid and an enzyme that digests protein. One of the unsolved puzzles of the digestive system is why the acid juice of the stomach does not dissolve the tissue of the stomach itself.

After the stomach empties the food and its juice into the small intestine, the juices of two other digestive organs, the pancreas and the liver, mix with the food to continue the digestion process. The pancreas produces an array of enzymes that break down carbohydrates, fat, and protein in food. Other enzymes involved at this stage of the process come from glands in the wall of the small intestine.

The liver produces bile, which is stored in the gallbladder until needed. At mealtime, the bile is squeezed out of the gallbladder through the bile ducts and into the intestine and mixes with the fat in our food. The bile acids dissolve the fat into the watery contents of the intestine, acting much like detergents that dissolve grease in water. Enzymes from the pancreas and the lining of the intestine digest the dissolved fat.

WHY USE HERBS?

Herbs' unique healing properties have a direct effect upon the lining of the alimentary canal. The herbs' constituents can directly touch the cells of the mucosa without first having to be assimilated into the bloodstream, travel through the liver, and make their way through the rest of the body before entering the cells from the blood. Thus, the body can rapidly reap the benefits of constituents that might reduce inflammation, relax muscles, combat bacterial infection, or promote the healing of wounds.

However, as with all true healing, any potential "cure" lies beyond the range of medicines, be they herbal or pharmaceutical. The healing process must involve a lifestyle change that includes a healthy diet and reduction of stress. Herbal medicine can bring about dramatic improvements in even profound digestive system problems, but you won't experience its full benefits unless you also follow a healthy lifestyle. The long-term maintenance of the benefits you get from herbs lies in your hands alone.

What Herbs Do

Europeans have long used herbs to aid digestion. From culinary herbs such as rosemary to "medicinal" alcohols such as vermouth or Chartreuse, Europeans use these remedies in large quantities. The very name "vermouth" is derived from the bitter remedy wormwood, whose name in German is *wermut*. In official pharmacopoeias, such as the *U.S. Pharmacopoeia* (USP) and *British Pharmacopoeia* (BP), herbs have the strongest foothold as therapeutic agents in the categories of digestive bitters, carminatives, and laxatives of varying strengths.

In the hands of a skilled herbalist, much can be achieved therapeutically. While each individual with a gastric ulcer, for example, will have his or her own set of unique causes, we can identify a treatment based on our knowledge of the different herbs.

Used holistically, herbal medicine offers specific remedies for particular pathological syndromes as well as preventive tonics and normalizers. Treating the problem within this context of general nurturing speeds improvement and reestablishes health and harmony.

Health and Wellness in the Digestive System

Ideally, we want to preserve health and maintain wellness rather than treat illness. Of course, there is much more to preventive medicine than simply taking "stuff" in the form of a medicinal plant or chemical drug. The World Health Organization (WHO) has a wonderful definition of health that helps put this idea in perspective: "Health is a state of complete physical, mental, and social well-being and not merely the absence of disease or infirmity."

Any attempt to promote wellness and prevent the development of disease must address the various complex factors that WHO identified. While this book cannot explore all of these factors in depth, it will help you identify a number of risk factors to minimize as well as positive actions to emphasize.

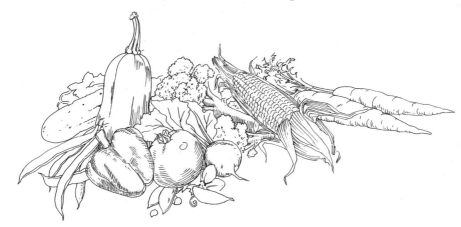

THE IMPORTANCE OF A GOOD DIET

By far the most important contribution we can make to the health of our digestive systems is the food we eat. Digestion makes all of the different nutrients available to the rest of the body. The human body requires over 40 nutrients for energy, growth, and tissue maintenance. All of these nutrients are found in a well-rounded diet, and many of them are found both in plants traditionally eaten as grains, vegetables, or fruits and those used as medicinal herbs. Often the only fundamental difference between a salad vegetable and a medicinal herb is that the vegetable tastes better!

Remember: Eating a balanced diet is a major factor in a healthy lifestyle. Using medicinal herbs does not eliminate the need for such a diet.

The official dietary guidelines, established jointly by the U.S. Departments of Agriculture and Health and Human Services, include seven basic recommendations:

- Eat a variety of foods. This will ensure you get enough calories, protein, and fiber as well as the vitamins, minerals, and other nutrients you need.
- Control your weight. Stay within recommended weight limits for your age, sex, and build. Obesity is defined as being 20 percent above ideal weight.
- Eat a low-fat, low-cholesterol diet. Ideally, no more than 30 percent of daily calories should come from fat and no more than 10 percent should come from saturated fat. Choose polyunsaturated fats over saturated fats whenever possible.
- Eat plenty of vegetables, fruits, and grains. They are rich in nutrients, fiber, and complex carbohydrates but low in fat. More than half of daily calories should come from carbohydrates, and 80 percent of these calories should come from complex carbohydrates.
- Eat sugar in moderation. Sugar is high in calories and also promotes tooth decay.
- Use salt in moderation. Consuming too much salt increases the risk of developing high blood pressure. Prepared foods are often high in salt or other forms of sodium.
- If you drink alcohol, do so in moderation. Alcohol provides calories but offers no nutrients, and too much alcohol is harmful.

If you consistently eat a well-balanced diet of fresh fruits, vegetables, grains, and some animal protein, you probably won't require a nutritional supplement. Multinutrient supplements offer insurance for those times when eating well is a challenge, and they can be indispensable during pregnancy and times of disease, injury, and extreme stress or physical exertion.

Water

Water, the most plentiful component in the body, is crucial to our survival. It is the medium for such bodily fluids as blood and lymph, and it transports nutrients into cells and carries out waste products and toxins. Most of the material absorbed from the cavity of the small intestine is water in which salt is dissolved. In a healthy adult, more than a gallon of water containing over an ounce of salt is absorbed from the intestine every 24 hours.

Carbohydrates

Carbohydrates, proteins, and fats — a dietary group known as macronutrients — provide fuel for the body in the form of calories. Carbohydrates, the body's main energy source, are divided into two types: simple carbohydrates, which are sugars; and complex carbohydrates, which are made up of sugars, fiber, and starches — such as those found in potatoes and bread. The average American adult eats about ½ pound of carbohydrates each day. Many of these carbohydrates consist of starch, which the body can digest, and fiber, which it can't digest. Enzymes in the saliva, in pancreatic juices, and in the lining of the small intestine break down the digestible carbohydrates into simpler molecules.

Proteins

Proteins support tissue growth and repair and help produce antibodies, hormones, and enzymes — which are essential for all chemical reactions in the body. Dietary protein sources include dairy products, beans, eggs, fish, meat, and nuts. An enzyme in the juice of the stomach starts the digestion of protein. Digestion is completed in the small intestine, where several enzymes in pancreatic juices and in the intestinal lining break huge protein molecules into small molecules called amino acids. These small molecules can be absorbed through the small intestine into the blood.

Fat

Dietary fat protects internal organs, provides energy, insulates against cold, and helps the body absorb certain vitamins. There are three kinds of fats: saturated, found in meat, dairy food, and coconut oil; monounsaturated, found in olive, peanut, and canola oils; and polyunsaturated, found in corn, cottonseed, safflower, soy, and sunflower oils. Bile acids produced by the liver dissolve fat in the watery content of the intestinal canal, allowing enzymes to break the large fat molecules into small molecules — some of which are fatty acids and cholesterol. In the mucosa, the small molecules are formed back into large molecules, most of which pass into the lymph vessels near the intestine.

Vitamins and Minerals

Your diet also supplies the important micronutrients we call vitamins and minerals. They are needed only in trace amounts, but the absence or deficiency of just one vitamin or mineral can cause major illness.

Vitamins and minerals are absorbed from the small intestine and passed into the bloodstream. There are two different types of vitamins, classified by the fluid in which they are dissolved: Water-soluble vitamins include all of the B vitamins and vitamin C, while the fat-soluble vitamins are A, D, E, and K.

Minerals fulfill a plethora of specific biochemical roles in the body, but they are especially important as essential components of enzymes and coenzymes. Without a balanced intake of minerals, the various digestive functions of the gut would be impaired.

Fiber

Dietary fiber is largely composed of the cellulose-like components of plant cell walls. Its composition is a complex of constituents and varies from plant to plant. This fiber is the part of fruits, vegetables, and grains that the body cannot digest. Soluble fiber dissolves easily in water, taking on a soft, jellylike texture in the intestines. Insoluble fiber passes almost unchanged through the intestines. Both kinds of fiber help make stools soft and easy to pass, preventing constipation. Since supplements lack this natural complexity, they cannot replace a varied diet rich in high-fiber foods.

Never underestimate the importance of dietary fiber. A high-fiber diet reduces the risks of various gastrointestinal problems and even promotes cardiovascular health. Here are some of fiber's benefits:

- Decreased intestinal transit time
- Delayed gastric emptying resulting in reduced after-meal elevations of blood sugar
- Increased satiety (feeling of "fullness")
- Increased pancreatic secretion
- Increased stool weight
- More soluble bile
- More beneficial intestinal microflora
- Increased production of short-chain fatty acids
- Decreased serum lipids

There is an abundance of research on the association between fiber and human health, and a number of conditions have been linked to low-fiber diets. In contrast, a high-fiber diet is associated with a decreased incidence of most of the degenerative diseases of Western society. Fiber alone is not a cure-all, but high-fiber diets also tend to be high in other nutrients — most of which are deficient in the "normal" Western diet.

The American Dietetic Association recommends we eat 20 to 35 grams of fiber each day. The best source of dietary fiber is whole foods, although specific types of fibers have their use in the treatment phase of specific diseases. There is no substitute for a healthy diet — that is, a diet composed of foods in a form as close to their original form as possible.

DIETARY FIBER CONTENT OF SELECTED FOODS

FOOD	SERVING SIZE	GRAMS OF FIBER
FRUITS		
Apple (with skin)	1 medium	3.5
Banana	1 medium	2.4
Cantaloupe	¼ melon	1.0
Cherries, sweet	10	1.2
Grapefruit	½ medium	1.6
Orange	1 medium	2.6
Peach (with skin)	1 medium	1.9
Pear (with skin)	½ large	3.1
Prunes	3	3.0
Raisins	¼ cup	3.1
Raspberries	½ cup	3.1
Strawberries	1 cup	3.0
VEGETABLES, RAW		
Bean sprouts	½ cup	1.5
Celery, diced	½ cup	1.1
Cucumber	½ cup	0.4
Lettuce	1 cup	0.9
Mushrooms	½ cup	1.5
Pepper, green	½ cup	0.5
Spinach	1 cup	1.2
Tomato	1 medium	1.5
VEGETABLES, COOKED		
Asparagus, cut	1 cup	2.0
Beans, green	1 cup	3.2
Broccoli	1 cup	4.4
Brussels sprouts	1 cup	4.6
Cabbage, red	1 cup	2.8
Carrots	1 cup	4.6
Cauliflower	1 cup	2.2
Corn	½ cup	2.9
Kale	1 cup	2.8
Parsnip	1 cup	5.4
Potato (with skin)	1 medium	2.5

Murray, Michael T., N.D. *The Encyclopedia of Nutritional Supplements,* © 1996 by Michael T. Murray. Reprint by permission of Prima Publishing, Roseville, CA.

(continued on next page)

DIETARY FIBER CONTENT OF SELECTED FOODS (cont'd)

	FOOD	SERVING SIZE	GRAMS OF FIBER
VEGETABLES, COOKED	Potato (without skin)	1 medium	1.4
	Spinach	1 cup	4.2
	Sweet potatoes	1 medium	3.4
	Zucchini	1 cup	3.6
LEGUMES	Baked beans	½ cup	8.8
	Dried peas, cooked	½ cup	4.7
	Kidney beans, cooked	½ cup	7.3
	Lentils, cooked	½ cup	3.7
	Lima beans, cooked	½ cup	4.5
	Navy beans, cooked	½ cup	6.0
BREADS, FLOUR, PASTAS, AND RICE	Bran muffins	1 muffin	2.5
	Bread, white	1 slice	0.4
	Bread, whole wheat	1 slice	1.4
	Crisp bread, rye	2 crackers	2.0
	Rice, brown, cooked	½ cup	1.0
	Rice, white, cooked	½ cup	0.2
	Spaghetti, regular, cooked	½ cup	1.1
	Spaghetti, whole wheat, cooked	½ cup	3.9
BREAKFAST CEREALS	All-Bran	⅓ cup	8.5
	Bran Chex	⅔ cup	4.6
	Corn Bran	⅔ cup	5.4
	Cornflakes	1¼ cup	0.3
	Grape-Nuts	¼ cup	1.4
	Oatmeal	¾ cup	1.6
	Raisin Bran	⅔ cup	4.0
	Shredded Wheat	⅔ cup	2.6
NUTS	Almonds	10 nuts	1.1
	Filberts	10 nuts	0.8
	Peanuts	10 nuts	1.4

BENEFICIAL EFFECTS OF DIETARY FIBER

Fiber can both help prevent and improve these conditions:

Cardiovascular conditions: cerebrovascular disease, deep vein thrombosis, hypertension, ischemic heart disease, pulmonary embolism, varicose veins

Colon conditions: appendicitis, colon cancer, constipation, Crohn's disease, diverticulitis, diverticulosis, hemorrhoids, irritable bowel syndrome, ulcerative colitis

Metabolic conditions: diabetes, gallstones, gout, kidney stones, obesity

Other conditions: autoimmune disorders, dental caries, dermatological conditions, multiple sclerosis, pernicious anemia, thyrotoxicosis

OTHER GOOD REASONS TO STOP SMOKING

In addition to causing heart and lung diseases, tobacco is responsible for changes in the digestive system. Smoking impacts all parts of the digestive system, contributing to such common problems as heartburn and peptic ulcers. Increases in the risk of Crohn's disease and possibly gallstones have also been connected with tobacco consumption.

Most of these effects on the digestive system appear to be of short duration, but a good piece of advice for digestive well-being is *stop smoking!*

Heartburn

Heartburn occurs when acidic juices from the stomach splash into the esophagus. Normally, a muscular valve at the lower end of the esophagus keeps the acid solution in the stomach. Smoking weakens this valve, allowing the stomach contents to flow backward into the esophagus. Smoking can also directly injure the esophagus, making it more prone to damage from refluxed material.

Peptic Ulcer

A peptic ulcer is an open sore in the lining of the stomach or duodenum, the first part of the small intestine. The exact cause of ulcers is not known, but the main cause is suspected to be bacterial infection. Some ulcers are caused by long-term use of nonsteroidal anti-inflammatory agents (NSAIDs), such as aspirin and ibuprofen. Occasionally, cancerous tumors in the stomach or pancreas can also cause ulcers. The 1989 Surgeon General's report stated that ulcers are more likely to occur, less likely to heal, and more likely to cause death in smokers than in nonsmokers.

Liver Disease

Among the liver's multitude of vital functions is the processing of drugs, alcohol, and other toxins to remove them from the body. Smoking alters the liver's ability to handle these substances. Some research also suggests that smoking can aggravate the course of liver disease caused by excessive alcohol intake.

Crohn's Disease

A severe gastrointestinal disorder that has no known cause, Crohn's disease produces inflammation deep in the lining of the intestine. The disease, symptoms of which are pain and diarrhea, usually affects the small intestine, but it can occur anywhere in the digestive tract. Both current and former smokers have a higher risk than nonsmokers of developing Crohn's disease. Smoking is associated with a higher rate of relapse, repeat surgery, and immuno-suppressive treatment.

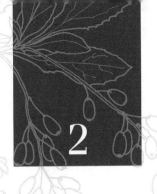

2

USING HERBS AS MEDICINE

The idea of using herbs as medicine goes back many centuries in many cultures. Unfortunately, in the early twentieth century most of Western society put aside herbal medicine in favor of allopathic treatments. But recently, interest in herbs has grown. We are now seeing a resurgence in herbal treatments for a variety of diseases.

THE ACTIONS OF HERBS

A great deal of pharmaceutical research has gone into analyzing the active constituents of herbs to find out how and why they work. However, a much older and far more relevant approach is to categorize herbs by the kinds of problems they can treat. In some cases the action is due to a specific chemical in the herb, while in other cases it might be due to a complex synergistic interaction between a number of the plant's constituents. It's always best to view the herb as a whole.

Because of its chemical complexity, a single herb might produce a range of responses in the body. For example, chamomile contains several active components in its volatile oil, in addition to nonvolatile flavonoids (aromatic compounds that frequently act as antioxidants and anti-inflammatories) and sesquiterpenes (hydrocarbon compounds). This cornucopia of chemistry allows chamomile to act as an anti-inflammatory, antispasmodic, antimicrobial, and relaxing nervine all in one!

Some herb constituents produce certain actions that are uniquely suited for treating digestive system problems. We group these actions into the following categories:

Adaptogens. Increase resilience and resistance to stress, enabling the body to avoid disease caused by overstress. Adaptogens appear to work by supporting the adrenal glands.

Alteratives. Gradually restore proper body function, increasing health and vitality. Some alteratives support natural waste elimination via the kidneys, liver, lungs, or skin. Others stimulate digestive function or are antimicrobial, while yet others just work — and we don't know why!

Analgesics. Relieve pain. The usual herbal approach to pain is to address the cause of the pain rather than block its experience.

Anticatarrhals. Help the body remove excess mucus, both in the sinus area and in other parts of the body. Excess mucus is usually produced in response to an infection or as a way of removing excess carbohydrates from the body.

Anti-inflammatories. Soothe or directly reduce inflammation. These herbs work in a number of ways but rarely inhibit the natural inflammatory reaction; rather, they support the body as it is working.

Antimicrobials. Help the body destroy or resist pathogenic microorganisms. While some antimicrobial herbs contain antiseptic chemicals or specific substances that are poisonous to certain organisms, in general they aid the body's natural immunity and help it throw off illness.

Antispasmodics. Ease muscle cramps and alleviate muscular tension. Many antispasmodic herbs are also nervines (see below), which ease psychological tension. Some antispasmodics reduce muscle spasming throughout the body, and others work on specific organs or systems.

Astringents. Have a bracing action on mucous membranes, skin, and other tissue. Astringents contain chemicals called tannins that help them bind with protein molecules, thus reducing irritation and inflammation and creating a barrier against infection. These herbs are helpful in healing wounds and burns.

Bitters. Trigger a sensory response in the central nervous system, which in turn sends a message to the gut telling it to release digestive hormones. These hormones stimulate appetite and the flow of digestive juices, aid the liver's detoxification work, increase bile flow, and stimulate self-repair mechanisms in the gut.

Cardiac remedies. Have a beneficial action on the heart. Some of the remedies in this group are powerful cardioactive agents, and others are gentler cardiotonics.

Carminatives. Stimulate the digestive system, soothe the gut wall, reduce inflammation, ease griping pains, and help remove gas from the digestive tract.

Cholagogues. Stimulate the flow of bile into the duodenum.

Demulcents. Soothe and protect irritated or inflamed tissue. Rich in mucilage, a gelatinous substance that consists mainly of carbohydrates, these herbs reduce irritation down the whole length of the bowel, reduce sensitivity to potentially corrosive gastric acids, help prevent diarrhea and reduce the muscle spasms that cause colic, ease coughing by soothing bronchial tension, and relax painful spasms of the bladder.

Diaphoretics. Promote perspiration, thus helping the skin eliminate waste from the body. Some diaphoretics produce observable sweat, while others aid normal perspiration. They often promote dilation of surface capillaries, which improves circulation. They support the work of the kidneys by increasing elimination through the skin.

Diuretics. Increase the production and elimination of urine. In herbal medicine, the term *diuretic* is often applied to herbs that have a beneficial action on the urinary system. They help the body eliminate waste and support the process of inner cleansing.

Emmenagogues. Stimulate menstrual flow and activity. The term *emmenagogue* is also applied to remedies that normalize and tone the female reproductive system.

Expectorants. Stimulate removal of mucus from the lungs and act as a tonic for the respiratory system. Stimulating expectorants "irritate" the bronchioles, causing expulsion of material. Relaxing expectorants soothe bronchial spasms and loosen mucus secretions, relieving dry, irritating coughs.

Galactogogues. Promote the secretion and flow of breast milk. (The opposite action, which decreases the flow, is known as a lactifuge.)

Hepatics. Aid the liver by toning, strengthening, and, in some cases, increasing the flow of bile. These herbs are of great importance because of the liver's fundamental role in the body.

Hypnotics. Help to induce a deep and healing state of sleep. These herbs have nothing at all to do with hypnotic trances!

Hypotensives. Lower abnormally elevated blood pressure.

Laxatives. Stimulate bowel movements. Laxatives should not be used long term; when constipation persists, closely consider diet, general health, and stress levels.

Nervines. Assist the nervous system. There are three types of nervines: Nervine tonics strengthen and restore the nervous system; nervine relaxants ease anxiety and tension by soothing both body and mind; and nervine stimulants directly stimulate nerve activity.

Tonics. Nurture and invigorate. Tonics truly are gifts of nature to a suffering humanity. To ask how they work is to ask how life works!

Vulneraries. Promote wound healing. The term *vulnerary* is used mainly to describe herbs that heal skin lesions, but the action is just as relevant for internal wounds, such as stomach ulcers.

Antispasmodics

Herbal antispasmodics, also called spasmolytics, prevent or ease spasms or cramps in the muscles. Many of the herbal remedies described as nervines, sedatives, or hypnotics also act as antispasmodics. General antispasmodics reduce muscle cramping throughout the body, while others work on specific organs or body systems. Antispasmodics relax the autonomic nervous system but not necessarily the central nervous system; in other words, they allow a physical relaxation of muscles without producing a sedative effect upon the mind.

When antispasmodic action is needed in the intestinal tract, carminative herbs often work exceedingly well. Since antispasmodics can be considered organ- or system-specific, it is important to select them based on the part of the body being treated. Here are some herbs that treat particular body systems:

- **Circulatory system** — black cohosh, cramp bark, lavender, lemon balm, motherwort
- **Digestive system** — barberry, chamomile, cramp bark, dill, fennel, hop, peppermint, sage, thyme, valerian, wild yam
- **Muscles and skeleton** — black haw, cramp bark, lobelia (used externally only), skullcap, valerian
- **Nervous system** — See Nervines (page 29) for more information.
- **Reproductive system** — black haw, cramp bark, skullcap, valerian
- **Respiratory system** — angelica, aniseed, garlic, grindelia, elecampane, lobelia, oregano, thyme, wild cherry, wild lettuce
- **Skin** — Antispasmodics are not directly relevant here.
- **Urinary system** — black haw, cramp bark, wild carrot

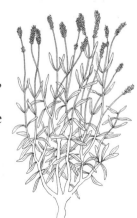

COMMON HERBAL ANTISPASMODICS

- Angelica
- Aniseed
- Black cohosh
- Black haw
- Caraway
- Cardamom
- Celery seed
- Chamomile
- Cramp bark

- Dill
- Fennel
- Fenugreek
- Feverfew
- Ginger
- Hop
- Hyssop
- Kava kava
- Lavender

- Lemon balm
- Licorice
- Linden
- Motherwort
- Mugwort
- Passionflower
- Peppermint
- Red clover
- Rosemary

- Skullcap
- St.-John's-wort
- Thyme
- Valerian
- Vervain
- Wild lettuce
- Wild yam

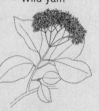

Intensity of Action in Antispasmodics
Knowing the strength of an herb's action is often important in choosing the appropriate treatment. Here is a guide to the intensity of different antispasmodic herbs.

Mild	Moderate	Strong
Angelica	Chamomile	Black cohosh
Aniseed	Feverfew	Black haw
Caraway	Ginger	Cramp bark
Cardamom	Hyssop	Hop
Celery seed	Lavender	Motherwort
Dill	Mugwort	Passionflower
Fennel	Red clover	Skullcap
Fenugreek	St.-John's-wort	Thyme
Lemon balm		Valerian
Linden		Vervain
Licorice		Wild lettuce
Peppermint		Wild yam
Rosemary		

Astringents

Saliva and other body fluids contain proteins that are soluble. Tannin-containing astringents cause those proteins to become insoluble and precipitate, or curdle. This action produces a coating — made of the body's own protein — that forms on the surface of tissue. Astringents won't cause allergic reactions, and because the precipitate is readily metabolized, their effect is short lived. Because their tannins come in direct contact with the tissue, astringents are most effective on damaged tissues of the mucosal lining of the gut.

Astringent herbs can be helpful for a wide range of problems but especially in wound healing

COMMON HERBAL ASTRINGENTS

• Agrimony	• Eyebright	• Periwinkle	• Witch hazel
• Bayberry	• Horse chestnut	• Plantain	• Yarrow
• Blackberry	• Kola nut	• Raspberry	
• Comfrey root	• Meadowsweet	• Red sage	
• Cranesbill	• Oak bark	• Rosemary	

Intensity of Action in Astringents
Knowing the strength of an herb's action is often important in choosing the appropriate treatment. Here is a guide to the intensity of different astringent herbs.

Mild	Moderate	Strong	Strong (continued)
Comfrey	Cranesbill	Agrimony	Raspberry
Plantain	Eyebright	Bayberry	Witch hazel
Red sage	Horse chestnut	Kola nut	
Rosemary	Meadowsweet	Oak bark	
	Yarrow	Periwinkle	

and conditions of the digestive system. These plants reduce inflammation and inhibit diarrhea. But long-term use of astringents can be harmful, as they can interfere with the absorption of food and nutrients.

Bitters

Bitter herbs are one of herbal medicine's great contributions to human health. Quite simply, this category contains herbs that have a bitter taste, ranging from mildly bitter yarrow to fiercely bitter rue. Absinthin, a constituent found in wormwood, is so bitter it can be tasted even at dilutions of 1 part in 30,000 parts of water. The strong flavor is often attributed to a "bitter principle," which can be a volatile oil, an alkaloid, an iridoid, or a sesquiterpene.

Following stimulation of the bitter receptors, located at the back of the tongue, a range of physiological responses occurs. Specific taste buds transmit the taste of bitterness to the central nervous system, triggering a number of reflexes. These reflexes have important ramifications, all of value to the digestive process and general health:

- The stimulation of the flow of digestive juices from the exocrine glands of the mouth, stomach, pancreas, duodenum, and liver aid in good digestion as well as helping a range of conditions caused by inefficient or allergy-distorted digestion.
- The flow of digestive juices triggers a stimulation of appetite. This is helpful in convalescence as well as in cases of appetite reduction.
- A range of liver activities is stimulated, including increased bile production and the release of bile from the gallbladder.
- A very mild stimulation of the endocrine glands occurs, producing insulin and glucagon secretions from the islets of Langerhans in the pancreas. Diabetics need to use bitters cautiously, as these herbs can change the blood sugar balance. In the hands of a skilled practitioner, however, bitter remedies

can play a role in the treatment of non–insulin-dependent diabetes.

- Bitter remedies can trigger subtle psychological effects, even acting as mild antidepressants. For example, bitters can help lift the spirits in cases of post–viral-infection depression.
- The central reflex stimulates peristalsis, an action that moves wastes through the intestines through a series of muscular contractions.
- Bitter remedies also stimulate the gut wall's self-repair mechanisms.

COMMON HERBAL BITTERS

- Barberry
- Boneset
- Chamomile
- Dandelion
- Gentian

- Goldenseal
- Hop
- Horehound
- Mugwort
- Rue

- Southernwood
- Tansy
- Wormwood
- Yarrow

Intensity of Action in Bitters
The strength of action is not particularly relevant in the case of bitters, but the subjective measure of taste approximates the physiological response a bitter herb might generate. Thus, we can identify mild and strong bitters, but to the bitter neophyte they might all seem strong!

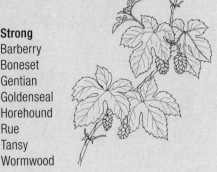

Mild	Strong
Chamomile	Barberry
Dandelion	Boneset
Mugwort	Gentian
Southernwood	Goldenseal
Yarrow	Horehound
	Rue
	Tansy
	Wormwood

Bitters' tonic effects go beyond the specifics of digestive hormone activity. Digestion and assimilation of food is fundamental to health, and bitter stimulation might improve a condition that has nothing, pathologically, to do with the digestive process.

There is much overlap in action between the bitters and tonics. The mechanism of their actions is not always clear, but it is evident that these herbs promote health — yet another wonderful gift of nature. Bitter stimulation effects are shared by any herb that can trigger the receptor sites on the tongue; consider each bitter's inherent strength, other actions, and specific indications to choose the most effective one.

Carminatives

Carminatives' main action is to soothe the gut wall, easing griping pains and reducing the production of gas in the digestive tract. A carminative herb's complex of volatile oils has local antispasmodic, anti-inflammatory, and mildly antimicrobial effects upon the lining and the muscle coats — layers of muscle that surround the mucous membranes of the gut — of the alimentary canal.

Although a carminative acts directly upon the intestinal tract, this leads to a more generalized effect on body systems. For exam-

COMMON HERBAL CARMINATIVES

• Angelica	• Eucalyptus	• Parsley
• Aniseed	• Fennel	• Pennyroyal
• Caraway	• Garlic	• Peppermint
• Cardamom	• Ginger	• Sage
• Celery seed	• Hop	• Thyme
• Chamomile	• Lemon balm	• Valerian
• Cinnamon	• Motherwort	• Wintergreen
• Dill	• Mustard	• Wormwood

ple, carminatives might occasionally ease what seem like symptoms of heart problems by removing the pressure of flatulence and digestive pain.

Cholagogues

Herbal cholagogues stimulate the flow of bile from the liver. In orthodox pharmacology there is a distinction between direct cholagogues, which actually increase the amount of bile the liver secretes, and indirect cholagogues, which simply increase the amount of bile the gallbladder releases. This difference is not very important in holistic herbal practice, especially since we are not going to use purified ox bile (an ingredient in many over-the-counter products and some "natural remedies")!

Most bitters and hepatics are also cholagogues. Many plant constituents have a bile-stimulating effect on the liver tissue, but they will not damage this important organ.

Without exploring the vast complexities of liver function, it's worth noting that bile formation and flow are fundamental to it all. We are what we eat — and we are also what we digest. Bile facilitates fat digestion, and since it is a natural laxative, it also cleanses the system. Thus, cholagogue herbs have a much deeper value than simply the release of bile; they help ensure a strong and healthy liver and, in doing so, enliven the whole being.

Cholagogues are used for:

- Long-term maintenance of impaired bile ducts, including stimulating normal contractions to deliver bile to the small intestine
- Disorders caused by insufficient or congested bile, such as intractable biliary constipation, jaundice, and nonviral hepatitis
- The treatment of autonomic functional disorders of the epigastric area (the anterior walls of the abdomen), including the symptoms of indigestion and the aiding of the digestion of fat-soluble substances

- Supporting the liver's detoxification work
- Gallstones, unless they are lodged in the bile duct and are causing a great deal of pain

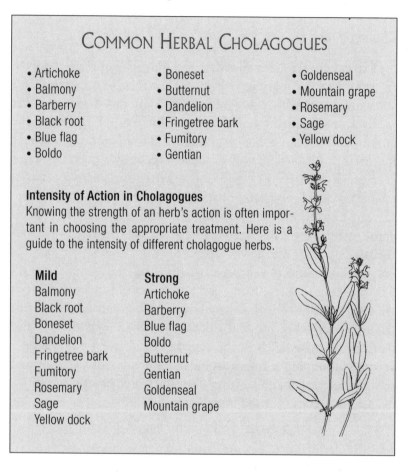

COMMON HERBAL CHOLAGOGUES

- Artichoke
- Balmony
- Barberry
- Black root
- Blue flag
- Boldo

- Boneset
- Butternut
- Dandelion
- Fringetree bark
- Fumitory
- Gentian

- Goldenseal
- Mountain grape
- Rosemary
- Sage
- Yellow dock

Intensity of Action in Cholagogues

Knowing the strength of an herb's action is often important in choosing the appropriate treatment. Here is a guide to the intensity of different cholagogue herbs.

Mild	Strong
Balmony	Artichoke
Black root	Barberry
Boneset	Blue flag
Dandelion	Boldo
Fringetree bark	Butternut
Fumitory	Gentian
Rosemary	Goldenseal
Sage	Mountain grape
Yellow dock	

Cholagogues should *not* be used for:

- Painful gallstones; the increased contractions could further constrict the bile duct, leading to incredibly intense pain
- Acute bilious colic
- Acute viral hepatitis

- Obstructive jaundice; the same reservations that apply to painful gallstones apply here
- Acute cholecystitis (inflammation of the gallbladder), unless gallstones have been ruled out; cholecystitis can be caused by infection, but a health care practitioner should determine the cause before you use a cholagogue
- Extremely toxic liver disorders; a cholagogue might be too stressful for a liver that is damaged to this extent, but you must weigh this against the potential benefits of the herb's liver-protecting properties

Demulcents

Demulcent herbs form protective barriers for irritated or inflamed tissue. When they are used on the skin, these herbs are called emollients. Because little research has been done, the action of demulcents cannot always be explained pharmacologically. They contain complex polysaccharide molecules of mucilage, which become slimy and gummy when in contact with water, soothing and reducing irritation in the lining of the intestines. The action of demulcents is actually quite passive, so one demulcent cannot be considered stronger than another.

> ### COMMON HERBAL DEMULCENTS
>
> - Comfrey
> - Corn silk
> - Couch grass
> - Flaxseed
> - Irish moss
> - Licorice
> - Marsh mallow
> - Mullein
> - Slippery elm

In general, demulcents:

- Reduce irritation down the whole length of the bowel
- Reduce the digestive system's sensitivity to gastric acids
- Help ease the digestive muscle spasms that cause colic

Some demulcents also ease coughing by soothing bronchial tension and relax painful spasms in the bladder, urinary system, and uterus.

Hepatics

Hepatics aid the work of the liver in a variety of ways. They tone, strengthen, and in some cases increase the flow of bile. The liver is well suited to herbal hepatic treatment because of the organ's fundamental role in the body.

In the unique language of traditional herbalists, much attention is given to "detoxifying the liver." Liver chemistry's incredible complexity and its important role in human physiology is so

---

COMMON HERBAL HEPATICS

- Agrimony
- Balmony
- Barberry
- Black root
- Bogbean
- Boldo
- Celery seed
- Dandelion

- Fennel
- Fringetree bark
- Fumitory
- Gentian
- Goldenseal
- Hyssop
- Lemon balm
- Milk thistle

- Motherwort
- Mountain grape
- Prickly ash
- Wild yam
- Wormwood
- Yarrow
- Yellow dock

Intensity of Action in Hepatics
Knowing the strength of an herb's action is often important in choosing the appropriate treatment. Here is a guide to the intensity of different hepatic herbs. There are a number of strong hepatics, but they are too powerful to be used without the supervision of an experienced herbalist. For this reason, this list is restricted to mild and moderate-strength hepatics.

Mild	Mild (continued)	Moderate	Moderate (continued)
Celery seed	Motherwort	Agrimony	Fringetree bark
Fennel	Prickly ash	Balmony	Gentian
Fumitory	Wild yam	Barberry	Goldenseal
Hyssop	Yarrow	Black root	Milk thistle
Lemon balm		Bogbean	Mountain grape
		Boldo	Wormwood
		Dandelion	Yellow dock

daunting to scientific researchers that the thought that simple plant remedies might have something to offer is laughable — even insulting! But these "common weeds" are proving to be superb tools in the treatment of liver diseases. For a more detailed look at the phytotherapeutic (or "plant therapy") approach to liver disease, see chapter 4.

There is no simple or single answer to the question of how hepatics work. Bitters and cholagogues all act as hepatics, but then so do a whole range of remedies without such specific actions. Hepatics are the epitome of an herbal remedy that does wonders for the body without its actions being fully understood.

Nervines

A nervine has a beneficial effect upon the nervous system. This makes "nervine" another catchall expression, so, in order to study them properly, it helps to separate nervines into a number of categories. Keep in mind that successful treatment of nervous system problems must involve treating the whole body, heart, and mind, not simply the *signs* of agitation and worry. After all, we can greatly reduce agitation, but we must strengthen the whole system in the face of the storm.

The main types of herbal nervines include:

Nervine tonics. Perhaps the most important contribution herbal medicine can make to the field of neurology is identifying those herbs that strengthen and "feed" the nervous system. In cases of shock, stress, or nervous debility, nervine tonics directly strengthen and restore the tissues. They also can contribute to the healing of trauma- or disease-damaged nerve tissue.

This invaluable group of remedies is best exemplified by oats, which are soothing, relaxing, and nutritious. An important tonic for the nervous system, ginkgo appears to work indirectly by dilating the blood vessels of the brain, which increases oxygen availability to brain cells. Some nervine tonics also have a relaxing effect; this group includes skullcap, St.-John's-wort, valerian, and vervain. Of these relaxing nervine tonics, skullcap is often the most effective, particularly for stress-related problems.

Nervine stimulants. Stimulating nervines, such as cola and guarana, directly arouse nervous tissue. Such direct stimulation is not often needed in today's hyperactive lifestyle. In most cases it is more appropriate to stimulate the body's innate vitality with the help of nervine tonics or bitters. In the past century, herbalists placed much more emphasis upon stimulant herbs. The change in this trend is, perhaps, a sign of the times — our world is supplying us with more than enough stimuli!

Nervine relaxants. These nervines are often important in times of stress and confusion, because they alleviate many of the accompanying symptoms. Nervine relaxants should always be used in a broad holistic way, not simply to tranquilize; too much tranquilizing, even from herbal medication, can in time deplete the nervous system. Many nervine relaxants also have other properties and can treat related problems. This is one of the great benefits of using herbal remedies to help ease stress and anxiety; we can treat the physical symptoms that so often accompany anxiety with herbs that also work to relieve the anxiety itself.

Some nervine relaxants are also antispasmodics, which affect peripheral nerves and muscle tissue and can have an indirect relaxing effect on the whole nervous system. When the body is at ease, it's easier for the psyche to relax. In addition to treating the nervous system, certain nervine relaxants benefit other body systems:

- **Circulatory system** — Lemon balm, linden, and motherwort are mild sedatives that reduce overactivity in the nervous system and, in doing so, aid heart function and treat problems such as high blood pressure.
- **Digestive system** — All of the antispasmodic remedies can ease colic, but sedatives that actively aid digestion include lemon balm, chamomile, hop, mugwort, lavender, valerian and vervain.
- **Musculoskeletal system** — All sedative remedies ease muscular tension and pain in this complex system. Remedies to bear in mind are black cohosh, cramp bark , kava kava, and wild yam.

COMMON NERVINE RELAXANTS

• Black cohosh	• Kava kava	• Red clover
• Black haw	• Lavender	• Skullcap
• California poppy	• Lemon balm	• St.-John's-wort
• Chamomile	• Linden	• Valerian
• Cramp bark	• Motherwort	• Vervain
• Hop	• Mugwort	• Wild lettuce
• Hyssop	• Passionflower	

Intensity of Action in Nervines

Knowing the strength of an herb's action is often important in choosing the appropriate treatment. Here is a guide to the intensity of different nervine herbs.

Mild	Moderate	Strong
Black haw	Black cohosh	California poppy
Chamomile	Motherwort	Hop
Cramp bark	Mugwort	Kava kava
Hyssop	Skullcap	Passionflower
Lavender	St.-John's-wort	Valerian
Lemon balm	Vervain	Wild lettuce
Linden		
Red clover		

- **Reproductive system** — Black cohosh, black haw, cramp bark, motherwort, and wild lettuce all benefit this system.
- **Respiratory system** — Most sedatives help in chest tension conditions such as asthma, but black cohosh, lobelia, motherwort, and wild lettuce are particularly valuable.
- **Skin** — Nervine relaxants might help the skin in an indirect way, but black cohosh, red clover, and St.-John's-wort all have a reputation for being beneficial to the skin.
- **Urinary system** — By relaxing the system, herbal nervine relaxants can encourage an increase in water loss. (This, however, does not make these herbs diuretics.) Nervine relaxants that benefit the urinary system include cramp bark, kava kava, and valerian.

REMEDIES FOR COMMON DIGESTIVE AILMENTS

Different conditions of the digestive system produce common processes, symptoms, and general experiences. Knowing herbal approaches that will address these general patterns helps the herbalist treat a specific disease.

Although herbal medicines alleviate the discomfort caused by specific diseases, treatment doesn't end there. The focus in phytotherapy, as in all holistic approaches to health, must go deeper than simply treating the symptoms. Learn as much as you can about your particular condition, and be sure you make any necessary lifestyle changes in addition to making herbal medicines part of your health regimen.

CONSTIPATION

This condition, which is a symptom rather than a disease, is defined as difficulty in passing or infrequent passage of feces. Correct diagnosis is vitally important.

Acute constipation is a definite, recognizable change that might be a sign of organic disease. With chronic constipation there is an ongoing hampering of normal bowel movements. In such cases, the ideal is to use diet to normalize and regularize bowel movements.

The most common cause of constipation in Western cultures is a lack of dietary fiber. However, there are some important, less common causes that the practitioner must bear in mind, ranging from irritable bowel syndrome, diverticular disease, and serious infection of the abdomen (e.g., appendicitis) to painful anal conditions that make the person afraid to open his or her bowels. Other causes include drugs that affect bowel motility, congenital diseases, endocrine disorders, diseases of the nervous system, diseases of the large intestine, and long periods of immobility, stress, or depression. A detailed discussion of these conditions is beyond the range of this book, but if you cannot determine which factor is the cause of your constipation you should seek advice from a qualified health care practitioner.

The "normal" size, frequency, and consistency of fecal output are difficult to quantify and are subject to personal variation and sociological patterning — the makers of laxatives take full advantage of this. There is no distinct benefit in having frequent bowel movements. While once-daily bowel movements might be average, a range from several times a day to once every several days is considered normal. If liver function is normal, fears of "autointoxication" by retention of colonic contents are unfounded.

The bulk, softness, and hydration of feces are very dependent on the fiber and water content of the diet. Dehydrated material can stay too long in the colon before expulsion, resulting in reduced colonic motility, frequency, and bulk and increased hardness of feces. Thus, sufficient dietary fiber and water are mainstays in any regimen for the treatment of constipation.

Treating with Herbs

Many herbs will alleviate the discomfort of constipation. Laxative remedies are obviously relevant, but we must consider other treatments as well. Because of their general stimulation of the digestive process, bitters can be very helpful. Where stress or depression is involved, consider the relaxing nervine, antispasmodic, and antidepressant herbs. Carminatives can also ease the pain and discomfort associated with constipation.

Effective herbs commonly used for constipation include yellow dock and psyllium seed. Anthraquinone is a substance that stimulates the nerve ganglia of the gut to activate peristaltic movement; a stronger combination of yellow dock and psyllium seed with anthraquinone-containing herbs such as senna might be appropriate in some cases. Of course, a dietary approach focusing on the rational use of fiber is the most effective treatment. I stress *rational* because becoming an oat bran supplement addict is not far from drug abuse!

Yellow Dock–Dandelion Tincture

This combination is a good general constipation reliever.

2 parts dandelion root
2 parts yellow dock
1 part aniseed

To make: Mix the herbs and make a tincture following the instructions on page 113.
To use: Take up to 1 teaspoon (5 ml) three times a day.

Using Laxatives

Laxatives promote defecation. The precise mechanisms by which they achieve results are unknown because of the complex factors that affect colonic function. Nevertheless, we can surmise three general mechanisms:

1. Laxatives may cause retention of fluid in colonic contents, thereby increasing bulk and softness and facilitating transit.

2. Laxatives may act, both directly and indirectly, on the colonic mucosa to decrease net absorption of water and salt.

3. Laxatives may increase intestinal motility, causing decreased absorption of salt and water secondary to decreased transit time. Reduced water absorption is a potential danger of laxatives.

A variety of laxatives are used to treat constipation:

Bulk laxatives are fiber-rich foods and herbs that are the only truly safe long-term treatments for constipation. These laxatives act slowly and gently and are best used through a gradual increase in dose, morning and evening, until a softer, bulkier stool results. Psyllium seed and whole wheat bread are examples of bulk laxatives.

Secretory laxatives stimulate bile production in the liver, thereby promoting bowel movement. Hepatics act as secretory laxatives.

Stimulant laxatives are herbs such as senna and cascara sagrada that contain anthraquinone. Stimulant laxatives should not be used long term.

Bulk Laxatives

Bulking and swelling agents are gentle laxatives that simulate the physiologic effects of a high-fiber diet; they can be used as supplements to dietary fiber. Bulk-forming agents are also widely recognized for their value in the long-term management of irritable colon and chronic diverticulitis. Examples of this type of laxative include polysaccharides and celluloses derived from grains, seed husks, or kelp, including bran, psyllium, methylcellulose, and carboxy-methylcellulose.

Bulking agents are normally components of food. Indigestible carbohydrates, which undergo complete or partial breakdown by the intestinal flora, physically stimulate activity through their bulking action, speeding the transit of material through the intestinal tract. Conversely, swelling agents are distinguished by their capacity to form mucilage or gels. Mucilaginous swelling agents are taken in some medicinal form (e.g., psyllium husks) rather than as foods per se. Like bulking agents, they are composed of indigestible carbohydrates; however, they undergo little or no degradation by intestinal flora. Bulk-forming laxatives in general have little effect on transit time through the small intestine, but they do affect colonic transit. The heavier the stool weight, the shorter the transit time.

More than 400 bacterial species inhabit the colon; their makeup is determined by the nature of the available substrate, or environment. Fecal bulk provides a substrate for bacterial proliferation, causing an increase in bacterial mass and stool weight. The bulk materials (celluloses, hemicelluloses, lignins, and pectins) contained in bulk-forming agents are not affected by human digestive enzymes, so they pass unchanged through the small intestine into the colon. There bacteria break down all or part of the bulk materials, releasing short-chain fatty acids, along with methane (in some people), carbon dioxide, and molecular hydrogen. Short-chain fatty acids promote the absorption of salts and water and stimulate bowel motility. Swelling agents soften the stool, enabling easier passage.

Gases generated in the lower bowel can cause bloating and flatulence, and bulking agents initially can worsen constipation. Generally this resolves once a new intestinal flora has been established. It might be useful to start treatment with half the normal bulk laxative dosage.

A CAUTION ON BULK-FORMING LAXATIVES

It is imperative to take all bulk-forming agents with sufficient liquid. After taking a bulk-forming laxative, intestinal obstruction and even impaction can occur, particularly in patients who have preexisting gastrointestinal disease; individuals with stenosis, ulceration, or adhesions of the large or small intestine should avoid these agents. Obstruction of the esophagus can also occur when these substances are ingested without adequate amounts of fluid.

Dietary Fiber

Dietary fiber is plant cell wall that is resistant to digestion by the secretions of the gastrointestinal tract. Sources of dietary fiber are whole grains, bran, vegetables, and fruits. Plant cell walls consist of varying quantities of fibrous polysaccharides (mainly cellulose), matrix polysaccharides (pectins, hemicelluloses), lignins, cutin, waxes, and some glycoproteins.

But foods differ widely in the type and amount of fiber they contain. Grains and cereals contain a preponderance of insoluble, poorly fermentable fibers; eating these will shorten intestinal transit time and increase stool bulk. Fruits and vegetables contain more water-soluble fibers, resulting in a moist stool but with less effect on transit time. Consuming 20 to 60 grams of dietary fiber daily usually is sufficient.

Dietary fiber acts as a laxative by:

- Binding water and ions in the colonic lumen (opening), thereby softening the feces and increasing their bulk. The water-binding capacity of fiber is, however, insufficient to combat the diarrhea that can be caused by materials excreted around blockages.
- Supporting the growth of colonic bacteria, thus increasing fecal mass.
- Being digested by colonic bacteria and broken down into metabolites, which contribute to laxative action by increasing the osmotic activity of the luminal fluid (the liquid inside the tube of the gut).
- Decreasing stool water. Colonic fermentation of the more water-soluble, noncellulose polysaccharides (such as pectins and gums) can decrease stool water, apparently by producing metabolites (such as short-chain fatty acids) that directly influence the colonic mechanisms of fluid and electrolyte transport.

Psyllium, lignin, and pectin bind bile acids, reducing the acids' intestinal reabsorption and promoting their excretion. This enhances hepatic synthesis of bile acids from cholesterol and can reduce plasma cholesterol in low-density lipoproteins. Over time, both dietary fiber and bulk-forming agents relieve the symptoms of irritable bowel syndrome and diverticular disease of the colon.

Osmotic Agents

Osmotic laxatives are chemicals that cause water to be retained in the bowel through osmosis, thus increasing the stool's water content. The action of nonabsorbable sugars, such as mannose, and sugar alcohols, such as mannitol and sorbitol, produce this effect.

Anthraquinone Laxatives

Many well-known laxative plants owe their efficacy to the presence of polyphenolic anthranoid compounds. These anthraquinone laxatives include 1,8-dihydroxyanthraquinone and its glycoside derivatives and are found in senna, cascara, rhubarb, aloe, and other members of the Liliaceae (lily) family.

Anthraquinones exert their laxative effect by damaging epithelial cells, leading to changes in the way nutrients are assimilated across the gut wall, in the activity of cells that secrete digestive juices, and in the way peristalsis moves material along the gut. Damaged epithelial cells can appear as dark patches in the colonic mucosa. This condition, called pseudomelanosis coli, is caused by chronic use of anthranoid laxatives and has recently been associated with an increased risk of colon and rectal cancer. In vitro and animal-human studies have shown a potential role of anthranoid laxatives in both the initiation and promotion of tumors. A 1999 study in humans also suggested tumor-promoting activities for these laxatives.

Although clinical evaluations of the long-term toxicity of anthraquinones are conflicting, preparations that contain 1,8-dihydroxyanthraquinone have been withdrawn from the market because of the chemical's association with hepatic and intestinal tumors in laboratory animals. Whether the naturally occurring glycosides have similar problems associated is not known.

Short-term use of anthraquinone laxatives is generally safe, but long-term use is not recommended. These laxatives may produce an excessive laxative effect and abdominal pain; large doses may produce nephritis (kidney inflammation). Most of the metabolites are excreted in the stool; however, a fraction is absorbed and appears in the urine, turning it a dark yellow or even red color. Do not use anthraquinone-containing herbs in association with:

> ### Fast Facts
>
> Senna is obtained from the dried leaflets or pods of *Senna alexandrina*. Cascara sagrada, or "sacred bark," is obtained from the bark of the buckthorn tree, *Rhamnus purshiana*.

• Partial or complete bowel obstruction
• Pregnancy
• Lactation

In addition, interactions with cardiac glycosides and other drugs can occur indirectly as a result of electrolyte imbalance.

Castor Oil

The bean of the castor plant, *Ricinus communis,* contains two well-known noxious ingredients: castor oil and the extremely toxic protein ricin. Used externally, castor oil is a bland emollient, but within the small intestine it causes the pancreatic enzymes to release ricinoleic acid. Ricinoleic acid and its salts reduce the absorption of fluid and electrolytes and stimulate intestinal peristalsis — and, hence, the movement of feces. Because it acts in the small intestine, accumulation of fluid and evacuation take place rapidly and are relatively complete. The cathartic effect is too strong to warrant using this agent for common constipation.

Uses and Abuses of Laxatives

In otherwise healthy people, laxatives are of secondary importance to a fiber-rich diet, adequate fluid intake, and appropriate physical activity. If constipation still develops, you can supplement with bulk-forming agents. Stimulant laxatives should be used only in unresponsive cases, and a qualified health care professional should supervise their use.

Take laxatives in the lowest effective dose, as infrequently as possible; discontinue their use promptly and completely upon termination of the need. If constipation is caused by medication, try changing the dosage or drug before using a laxative.

In addition to perpetuating dependence on drugs, the laxative habit can lead to serious gastrointestinal disturbances, such as irritable bowel syndrome, and other functional ills have been associated with the habitual use of stimulant laxatives. Always remember that constipation is a symptom of a disease, and the use of laxatives is no substitute for treating the underlying problem. Laxatives can be used safely to:

- Soften feces
- Prevent straining during defecation (especially in the elderly and in people with cardiac disease or hernia)
- Evacuate the bowel prior to diagnostic or surgical procedures

Laxatives are often useful, both before and after surgery, to maintain soft feces in patients with hemorrhoids and other anorectal disorders. For these purposes, dietary fiber or the bulk-forming agents are generally satisfactory and preferable. A fiber-rich diet and specific pharmaceutical drugs also have an established role in the management of diverticular disease of the colon and irritable bowel syndrome.

DIARRHEA

Like constipation, diarrhea is an important symptom that can have many causes. These range from intestinal infection and food sensitivities to colitis and anxiety. Again, accurate diagnosis is essential, and simply alleviating the symptom can be dangerous.

Technically, diarrhea is loose, watery stools occurring more than three times in one day. It is a common problem that usually lasts a day or two and goes away on its own without any special treatment. However, prolonged diarrhea can be a sign of other, more serious problems.

Diarrhea can be a temporary or a chronic problem. A few of the more common causes of diarrhea are:

- **Bacterial infections.** Several types of bacteria, consumed through contaminated food or water, can cause diarrhea. Common culprits include *Campylobacter, Escherichia coli, Salmonella,* and *Shigella.*
- **Viral infections.** Many viruses cause diarrhea, including cytomegalovirus, herpes simplex virus, Norwalk virus, rotavirus, and the hepatitis viruses.
- **Food intolerance.** One example is lactose intolerance, the inability to digest the sugar found in milk.
- **Parasites.** Those that cause diarrhea include *Cryptosporidium, Entamoeba,* and *Giardia.*
- **Reaction to medicines,** such as antibiotics, blood pressure medications, and antacids containing magnesium.
- **Intestinal diseases,** such as inflammatory bowel disease.
- **Functional bowel disorders,** such as irritable bowel syndrome, in which the intestines do not work normally.

Diarrhea can be accompanied by cramping pain, bloating, nausea, fever, bloody stools, or an urgent need to use the bathroom. Acute diarrhea lasts less than three weeks and is usually related to an infection. Chronic diarrhea lasts longer than three weeks and is often related to functional disorders. The chronic diarrhea of colitis is treated differently from "Delhi Belly" or its New World relative "Montezuma's Revenge."

Although usually not harmful, diarrhea might be a sign of a more serious problem. You should see a professional if:

- The diarrhea lasts for more than three days.
- There is severe pain in the abdomen or rectum.
- A fever of 102°F (39°C) or higher develops.
- There is blood in the stools or the stools become black and tarry.
- You show signs of dehydration.

Diarrhea can cause dehydration, meaning that the body will lack the fluid needed to function properly. Dehydration is particularly dangerous in children and the elderly and must be treated

DIARRHEA IN CHILDREN

The dehydrating effects of diarrhea are potentially dangerous in newborns and infants. Signs of dehydration in children include:

- No wet diapers for 3 hours or more
- Sunken abdomen, eyes, or cheeks
- Listlessness or irritability
- Dry mouth and tongue
- Lack of tears when crying
- High fever
- Skin that does not flatten when pinched and released

The fluid and electrolytes (especially potassium and sodium) lost through diarrhea must be replaced, as the body cannot function properly without them. Along with water, give your child a commercial dehydration solution (available at any pharmacy) that contains the electrolytes and nutrients needed.

Take your child to the doctor if signs of dehydration or any of the following symptoms appear:

- Stools containing blood or pus, or black stools
- Temperature above 101.4ºF (38ºC)
- No improvement after 24 hours

promptly to avoid serious health problems. General signs of dehydration include thirst, infrequent urination, dry skin, fatigue, and light-headedness. Water is essential in preventing dehydration, but it does not contain the electrolytes the body needs. To maintain electrolyte levels, you should also have chicken, beef, or vegetable broth, which contain sodium, and fruit drinks, which contain potassium.

Treating with Diet

In most cases, replacing the lost fluids to prevent dehydration is the only treatment necessary. Medicines that stop diarrhea might be helpful in some cases, but they are not recommended when the diarrhea is caused by bacterial or parasitic infection; the medications stop the diarrhea, trapping the organism in the intestines and prolonging the problem.

Until diarrhea subsides, try to avoid dairy products and foods that are greasy, high in fiber, or very sweet; these types of food tend to aggravate diarrhea. When the diarrhea begins to improve, add soft, bland foods — including bananas, plain rice, boiled potatoes, toast, crackers, cooked carrots, and baked chicken without the skin or fat — to your diet. For children, pediatricians recommend what is called the BRAT diet: bananas, rice, applesauce, and toast.

Treating with Herbs

It is difficult to say whether astringent herbs are specific remedies for diarrhea, or whether they are simply good examples of the general effect of astringency.

Meadowsweet may well be the best gentle treatment for diarrhea in general, as it seems to tone the lining of the small intestine. It is especially helpful in childhood diarrhea. Other excellent remedies include agrimony, cranesbill, and lady's mantle. The stronger astringents, such as oak bark, should be used only when the gentler ones prove ineffective.

Simple Diarrhea Infusion

This formula is designed to ease the general symptoms of diarrhea.

1 part agrimony	1 part cranesbill
1 part chamomile	

To make: Mix the herbs and make an infusion following the instructions on page 109.

To use: Drink regularly (approximately every hour) throughout the day until symptoms subside.

DIVERTICULITIS

Diverticula are small saclike herniations or pouches of the mucosal lining of the colon that bulge outward through weak spots in the colon wall. About half of all Americans age 60 to 80, and almost everyone over age 80, have these herniations, a condition called diverticulosis. The condition is also found in 30 to 40 percent of people over the age of 50.

When diverticula become inflamed or infected, the condition is called diverticulitis. This happens in 10 to 25 percent of people with diverticulosis. It is thought that a highly refined low-fiber diet is a primary cause of the condition. Diverticulitis is common in industrialized countries where low-fiber diets are usual, but it is rare in countries where people eat high-fiber vegetable diets. The ailment was first noticed in the United States in the early 1900s, the time when processed foods were introduced. Many processed foods contain refined, low-fiber flour, which (unlike whole wheat flour) contains no bran.

Constipation causes muscles to strain if the stool is too hard, increasing pressure in the colon. The pressure causes weak spots in the colon to bulge out. An attack of diverticulitis can develop suddenly and without warning.

The most common sign of diverticulitis is tenderness around the left side of the lower abdomen. If infection is the cause, fever, nausea, vomiting, chills, cramping, and constipation alternating with diarrhea can occur as well. The severity of symptoms depends on the extent of the infection and complications. Bleeding from diverticula is rare, but if it occurs blood might appear in the toilet or in your stool. Bleeding can be severe, but it might stop by itself. Nonetheless, if you have bleeding from the rectum, you should see a doctor. A professional diagnosis is essential to rule out colon cancer.

Lifestyle Treatments

Diverticular disease appears to be associated with a low-fiber diet, and there is little doubt that most patients gain some relief when they switch to a high-fiber diet. The underlying bowel abnormality remains, but it does not cause the same degree of problems.

When the symptoms are acute and severe, a low-fiber diet is called for initially to ensure that roughage does not cause physical irritation. This is especially the case in people who are not used to a high-fiber diet. As soon as the discomfort is brought under control, the proportion of fiber can be increased gradually.

Treating with Herbs

Wild yam is a very useful specific remedy for diverticulitis. It is a good general antispasmodic and anti-inflammatory, but it has a quite specific impact upon this condition by easing the chronic spasming colic pain that characterizes diverticulitis. You must take care not to induce constipation through overuse of astringent herbs. In general:

- Antispasmodics will help relieve pain caused by abdominal cramping around the diverticula.
- Carminatives relieve discomfort due to flatulence.

- Anti-inflammatories ease generalized inflammation within the colon.
- Antimicrobials help the body deal with any infection that might be present.
- Nervines ease the stress involved, which can be a cause or result of the condition.
- An infusion of chamomile or peppermint sipped slowly throughout the day will help. Add garlic to the diet, raw (one clove a day) or as a supplement in capsule form.

Diverticulitis Tincture

This formula supplies the range of actions needed to relieve diverticulitis, including antispasmodic (cramp bark, peppermint, wild yam), anti-inflammatory (peppermint, wild yam), antimicrobial (garlic), carminative (peppermint, valerian), and nervine (peppermint, valerian) actions. An infusion of chamomile or peppermint sipped throughout the day will support the work of the tincture.

2 parts wild yam	1 part peppermint
1 part cramp bark	1 part valerian

To make: Mix the herbs and make a tincture following the instructions on page 113.
To use: Take up to 1 teaspoon (5ml) three times a day for at least one month.

FLATULENCE

Everyone produces gas and eliminates it by burping or passing it through the rectum. The average person produces 1 to 3 pints a day and passes gas at least 14 times a day. Most people do not realize that passing gas 14 to 23 times a day is normal.

Gas is made primarily of odorless vapors — carbon dioxide, oxygen, nitrogen, hydrogen, and sometimes methane. The unpleasant odor of flatulence comes from bacteria in the colon that release small amounts of sulfur-containing gases. This intestinal gas comes from two different sources: swallowed air, or the breakdown of undigested foods by the bacteria that are naturally present in the colon.

Air swallowing, or aerophagia, is a common cause of gas in the stomach. We all swallow some air when eating and drinking; however, eating or drinking rapidly, chewing gum, smoking, or wearing loose dentures can lead to the intake of more air. Burping is the usual way air leaves the stomach, but any remaining gas moves into the small intestine where it is partially absorbed. A small amount travels into the large intestine for release through the rectum.

FOODS THAT CAN CAUSE GAS

- Beans
- Vegetables, such as artichokes, asparagus, broccoli, brussels sprouts, cabbage, and onions
- Fruits, such as apples, peaches, and pears
- Whole grains, such as whole wheat
- Bran
- Soft drinks and fruit drinks
- Milk and milk products, such as cheese and ice cream, and packaged foods prepared with lactose, such as bread, cereal, and salad dressing
- Foods containing sorbitol, such as dietetic foods and sugar-free candies and gums

The body does not digest and absorb some carbohydrates in the small intestine, because certain enzymes that are absent in this organ are necessary for this action. Undigested food passes into the large intestine, where bacteria might break it down, producing the gases hydrogen, carbon dioxide, and, in about one-third of all people, methane. Research has not determined why some people produce methane and others do not.

Lifestyle Treatments

Foods containing carbohydrates can cause gas, but fats and proteins cause little gas. What's more, foods that produce gas in one person might not cause it in another.

Sugars. The sugars that cause gas include fructose, lactose, raffinose, and sorbitol:

- Fructose is naturally present in artichokes, onions, pears, and wheat. It is also used as a sweetener in some soft drinks.
- Lactose, the sugar in milk, is found in all milk-based products, such as cheese and ice cream. Processed foods, such as bread, cereal, and salad dressing, also contain lactose. Many people have low levels of the enzyme lactase that is needed to digest lactose. As people age, their lactase levels may decrease.
- Raffinose is present in beans in large amounts. Smaller amounts are found in asparagus, broccoli, brussels sprouts, cabbage, other vegetables, and whole grains.
- Sorbitol is a sugar found naturally in fruits, including apples, pears, peaches, and prunes.

Starches. Most starch sources, such as potatoes, corn, noodles, and wheat, produce gas as they are broken down in the large intestine. Rice is the only starch that does not cause gas.

Fiber. Soluble fiber dissolves easily in water and takes on a soft, gel-like texture in the intestines. Found in beans, oat bran, peas, and most fruits, soluble fiber does not break down until it reaches the large intestine, where the digestion process causes gas. Insoluble fiber, on the other hand, passes essentially unchanged through the intestines and produces little gas. Wheat bran and some vegetables contain this type of fiber.

Treating with Herbs

Flatulence is a common problem that can be associated with a pathology or can simply be related to an inappropriate diet. The production of excessive gas by the digestive system has many causes, so it is best to think in general terms about the relevant actions of different plants. The green world abounds in herbs that can alleviate the discomfort of flatulence.

In flatulence, the processes at work are very closely interrelated. Inflammation of the lining of the intestinal tract will usually lead to flatulence, but as with all inflammation, it is important to identify the cause. Of the range of anti-inflammatory herbs available to the herbalist, those containing volatile oils are the best choices. Inflammation and flatulence can also be caused by some variety of infection, making antimicrobials a relevant treatment.

You should also consider problems with digestion and possible malabsorption. In these cases, the use of bitters is indicated. Where muscular cramping in the gut or anxiety and tension are involved, consider both the nervine and antispasmodic herbs. Carminatives are a good place to start, but bitters will be more useful for digestive problems.

We are blessed with a group of herbs that actually possess most of these actions. They are known as carminatives, and most

Flatulence Relief Tea

Use this mild remedy whenever flatulence becomes problematic.

Lemon balm
Chamomile

To make: Mix equal parts lemon balm and chamomile, and make an infusion as instructed on page 109.
To use: Drink a warm cup of the tea at regular intervals until symptoms subside.

of the commonly used culinary and mild medicinal herbs have this property. Well-known examples are lemon balm, chamomile, marjoram, peppermint, and sage. See page 24 for more information on carminatives.

GASTRITIS

Strictly speaking, the term *gastritis* means inflammation of the gastric mucosa, the tissue lining the stomach. But there is a range of subdivisions of this ailment based upon the various pathological changes that might have occurred to the tissue. From the herbal perspective, however, these findings are not crucial. You can apply the approach described here in all cases unless there is another problem more pressing than the gastritis.

Heartburn, also called acid indigestion, is the most common symptom of gastritis; it usually feels like a burning chest pain beginning behind the breastbone and moving upward to the neck and throat. Heartburn pain can be mistaken for the pain associated with heart disease or a heart attack, but there are differences. Exercise might aggravate pain resulting from heart disease, and rest can relieve the pain. Heartburn pain is less likely to be associated with physical activity.

Lifestyle Treatments

Lifestyle is fundamental to both the cause and treatment of gastritis. If you suffer from heartburn, you must avoid food irritants, which include chemicals, extremely hot or cold foods/drinks, and fiber (during acute attacks only). Avoid acid foods, such as citrus or vinegar, alcohol, tobacco, and anything that elicits the symptoms. Stress will aggravate and can even cause gastritis; consider work conditions, relationships, anxiety level, and other personal factors. (You'll find a more complete discussion of these personal factors under Peptic Ulceration on page 67.)

Antacids temporarily relieve the symptomatic discomfort of gastritis by lessening stomach acidity. But these substances have little to offer in terms of actual healing, as the body will compensate for their effects by increasing the secretion of hydrochloric acid.

Treating with Herbs

Appropriate herbal treatment of gastritis begins with identifying what actions might be indicated for the processes involved in the condition. With gastritis, the inflammation is a primary focus in deciding upon relevant actions and herbs. A number of herbs will reduce the inflammation, but they do not replace any necessary dietary or lifestyle changes.

The primary options are using demulcents as a barrier between the acidic stomach content and the inflamed tissues and using anti-inflammatories to lessen the inflammatory response within the cells. Simple demulcents are usually quite adequate, as

---

Soothing Gastritis Remedy

This tincture combines demulcents (comfrey root, marsh mallow root), an anti-inflammatory (chamomile), and a nervine (chamomile) for maximum effect. Sip a cold infusion of marsh mallow root throughout the day to support the work of the tincture.

2 parts comfrey root
2 parts marsh mallow root
1 part chamomile

To make: Mix the herbs and make a tincture following the instructions on page 113.
To use: Take up to 1 teaspoon (5 ml) three times a day.

the body will do the healing work itself, given the chance. Sip a cold infusion of marsh mallow root often throughout the day. Use relaxing nervines if stress and anxiety are involved.

GASTROESOPHAGEAL REFLUX

This relatively common and unpleasant problem affects the lower esophageal sphincter (LES), the muscular valve connecting the esophagus with the stomach. The condition is technically called gastroesophageal reflux disease (GERD); *gastroesophageal* refers to the stomach and esophagus, and *reflux* means "to flow back." The name is an apt description for the condition, in which the stomach's contents flow back up into the esophagus, causing heartburn or acid indigestion.

Normally the LES valve opens to allow food to pass into the stomach and closes to prevent food and acidic stomach juices from flowing back into the esophagus. GERD occurs when the valve is weak or relaxes inappropriately, allowing the stomach's contents to flow up into the esophagus. The severity of GERD depends on LES dysfunction as well as the type and amount of fluid brought up from the stomach and the neutralizing effect of the saliva.

Heartburn is GERD's main symptom, and it feels like a burning pain beginning behind the breastbone and moving upward to the neck and throat. It might feel like food is coming back into the mouth, leaving an acid or bitter taste. This can last as long as two hours and is often worse after eating. Lying down or bending over can also result in heartburn. Heartburn pain can be mistaken for the pain associated with heart disease or a heart attack, but there are differences. For instance, exercise can aggravate pain resulting from heart disease, and rest can relieve the pain. Heartburn pain is less likely to be associated with physical activity.

Lifestyle Treatments

Dietary and lifestyle choices contribute to GERD. Certain foods and beverages, including chocolate, peppermint, fried or fatty foods, coffee, and alcoholic beverages, can weaken the LES, causing reflux and heartburn. Cigarette smoking also relaxes the valve. Another major cause is a structural weakness of the diaphragm, called a hiatal hernia. Obesity and pregnancy can also cause GERD. And, while stress does not cause GERD, it compounds it greatly.

Lifestyle and dietary changes are effective for most people. Treatment aims at decreasing the amount of reflux or reducing the damage to the lining of the esophagus from refluxed materials. Following this simple advice will reduce much of the discomfort while also treating the underlying problem:

- Raise the head of the bed. This reduces heartburn by allowing gravity to minimize reflux of stomach contents into the esophagus.
- Avoid stooping and constricting pressure on the abdomen (such as that caused by very tight clothes).
- Avoid foods and beverages that can weaken the LES. These foods include chocolate, peppermint, fatty foods, coffee, and alcoholic beverages. Also avoid foods and beverages that can irritate a damaged esophageal lining, such as citrus fruits and juices, tomato products, and pepper.
- Decrease the size of portions at mealtime and eat meals at least two to three hours before bedtime. These measures can lessen reflux by allowing the acid in the stomach to decrease and the stomach to empty partially.
- Stop smoking. Cigarette smoking weakens the LES; quitting will help reduce GERD symptoms.
- Deal with — don't ignore — stress, anxiety, and any systemic health problems.

Antacids neutralize acid in the esophagus and stomach and stop heartburn. Nonprescription antacids provide temporary relief, but avoid their long-term use, as it can lead to diarrhea, altered calcium metabolism, and buildup of magnesium in the body. Too much magnesium can be serious for patients with kidney disease. In addition, since most commercial antacids contain peppermint, some people may respond to them with GERD-like symptoms.

Treating with Herbs

Specific remedies will not replace a balanced prescription that takes into account the individual's needs. The entire digestive system must be helped, as the disruption of stomach function can lead to problems with digestion and assimilation of nutrients. And stress is involved, whether it's the cause or a result of the condition. Nevertheless, several herbs are used for treating GERD:

- Demulcent herbs such as marsh mallow soothe and coat the tissue of the esophagus, insulating the tissue lining from acidic stomach contents.
- Anti-inflammatories such as calendula, chamomile, and lemon balm will reduce any localized mucosal reaction.
- Vulneraries such as calendula and comfrey aid the natural healing process of ulcerations and other lesions.
- Astringents such as meadowsweet will lessen any minor local ulcer bleeding.
- Carminatives, such as chamomile, might be needed if there is a more general disruption of the digestive process.

Note: Bitters are contraindicated, because they stimulate the secretion of stomach acid as well as peristaltic activity.

A cold infusion of marsh mallow root sipped slowly throughout the day will minimize symptomatic discomfort.

Marsh Mallow Soother

This combination supplies a demulcent (marsh mallow); lymphatic vulnerary astringent (calendula); anti-inflammatory (chamomile and calendula); and carminative (chamomile).

2 parts marsh mallow root
1 part calendula
1 part chamomile flowers

To make: Mix the herbs and make a tincture following the instructions on page 113.
To use: Take up to 1 teaspoon (5 ml) three times a day.

INDIGESTION (FUNCTIONAL DYSPEPSIA)

Indigestion, also known as upset stomach or dyspepsia, is a painful or burning feeling in the upper abdomen, often accompanied by nausea, abdominal bloating, belching, and sometimes vomiting.

Indigestion might be caused by a disease, but for most people it results from eating too much, eating too quickly, eating high-fat foods, or eating during stressful situations. Smoking, drinking alcohol, using medications that irritate the stomach lining, being tired, and experiencing ongoing stress can also aggravate or cause indigestion. This is a vague and variable problem that is functional in nature and usually does not have an underlying structural cause.

Belching, distension, and borborygmus (rumbling in the intestines) often occur, associated with abdominal or epigastric pain. Frequently cases of indigestion have an overt psychological component, but it is incorrect to conclude that all indigestion is psychosomatic. Other symptoms of indigestion include signs of cardiac ischemia (obstruction of oxygen flow to heart tissues), peptic ulceration, and cholecystitis (inflammation of the gallbladder, see page 77 for more information). Differential diagnosis is crucial. Any case of indigestion that does not improve needs the immediate attention of a health care professional.

Lifestyle Treatments

Persistent indigestion calls for skilled medical diagnosis. Because of the functional nature of this problem, just about anything that eases discomfort or improves your physiological activity will be indicated. Diet is fundamental. Therapies from chiropractic adjustment to rolfing to psychological counseling often help.

Avoiding the foods and situations that seem to cause indigestion is the most successful way to treat it. Excess stomach acid does not cause or result from indigestion, so antacids are not an appropriate treatment — although some people report that they do help. Smokers can help relieve their indigestion by quitting smoking or at least not smoking right before eating. Exercising with a full stomach can cause indigestion, so scheduling exercise for before a meal or at least an hour afterward might help.

Because indigestion can be a sign of, or mimic, a more serious disease, consult a doctor if you experience:

• Vomiting, weight loss, or appetite loss
• Black, tarry stools or bloody vomit
• Severe pain in the upper right abdomen
• Discomfort unrelated to eating
• Shortness of breath, sweating, or pain radiating to the jaw, neck, or one of the arms

Treating with Herbs

The key to correcting functional dyspepsia is "tuning up" the fine control of both metabolic and physical aspects of digestion and assimilation while also easing the discomfort with appropriate remedies. For herbal remedies, it's important to know that:

- Bitter stimulation will promote digestive secretions in response to food or hunger as well as increasing muscular tone in peristalsis.
- Carminatives will ease flatulence, reduce localized inflammation and muscular spasm leading to colic, and act as mild antimicrobials.
- Antispasmodics might be indicated if the carminatives do not ease abdominal cramping.
- Nervines can be used to help ease stress, anxiety, and tension. They are usually also antispasmodic.

Every herbalist and every culture has favorite remedies for indigestion. These are often bitter carminatives or nervine carminatives. European specific remedies include lemon balm, chamomile, gentian, hop, peppermint, and valerian.

Combination Indigestion Tincture

You can augment the Indigestion Simple (opposite) with a combination of tinctures that aid the digestive system in general through a bitter/carminative approach.

Chamomile tincture
Gentian tincture
Peppermint tincture
Valerian tincture

Combine equal parts of the tinctures, up to ½ teaspoon (2.5ml) total, and take 10 minutes before each meal.

Indigestion Simple

The traditional simple, or tea made from a single fresh remedy, is best for correcting indigestion. Use an herb whose taste and aroma you like. Ideally, choose a plant you can easily cultivate, thus providing a steady supply of fresh leaves.

Chamomile, lemon balm, or peppermint

To make: Mix the herbs and make an infusion following the instructions on page 109.

To use: Drink a cup either just before or after meals; experiment to see which time produces the best effect.

A COMBINATION APPROACH

Using the indigestion tea and tincture formulas in conjunction will provide:
- Anti-inflammatories (chamomile, lemon balm, peppermint)
- Bitters (chamomile, gentian)
- Carminatives (chamomile, lemon balm, peppermint)
- Nervines (chamomile, valerian)

INFLAMMATORY BOWEL DISEASE

Inflammatory bowel disease is the term used to describe two chronic intestinal disorders: Crohn's disease and ulcerative colitis. IBD affects between 2 and 6 percent of Americans (300,000 to 500,000 people). The causes of both Crohn's disease and ulcerative colitis are not known, but both are often considered immune conditions in which the body's immune response alters, triggering an inflammatory reaction in the intestinal wall. The onset for both diseases occurs in young adulthood.

Either disease can cause persistent abdominal pain, bowel sores, diarrhea, fever, intestinal bleeding, and weight loss. Inflammatory bowel disease usually presents as a series of attacks of bloody diarrhea varying in intensity and duration. These will alternate with periods of no symptoms at all. Note that blood in the stools is *always* a sign that skilled diagnosticians must investigate further.

Lifestyle Treatments

Nutrition is a crucial issue in IBD, as there is often some degree of malabsorption. There are a number of contributing factors behind this nutritional deficit, each of which indicates the need for a specific therapy. These factors include:

- **Decreased food intake** due to pain, diarrhea, nausea, anorexia, or therapeutic dietary restrictions
- **Malabsorption** because of decreased absorptive surface due to disease or surgery; bile salt deficiency following surgery; bacterial flora overgrowth; or drugs such as corticosteroids, sulfasalazine, and cholestyramine
- **Increased secretion and nutrient loss** due to protein-losing enteropathy (a condition in which plasma protein is lost); or electrolyte, mineral, and trace mineral loss in diarrhea
- **Increased utilization and increased energy requirements** due to inflammation, fever, infection, or increased intestinal cell turnover

A good multivitamin and mineral supplement will help. In the *Textbook of Natural Medicine,* Pizzorno and Murray recommend vitamin supplementation in amounts of at least five times the U.S. recommended daily amount (RDA). Important minerals in treating IBD are zinc, magnesium, and, where there is loss of blood via the gut, iron. Electrolyte replacement is recommended if there is much diarrhea.

Initially, you should avoid high fiber to minimize irritation of the inflamed mucosa; as the symptoms are brought under control, increase the amount of fiber. Lactobacillus-rich yogurt is most helpful.

Treating with Herbs

More than in any of the conditions discussed in this book, a skilled herbalist is a necessity in treating inflammatory bowel disease effectively with herbs. The suggestions here are not meant to replace a balanced prescription that takes into account the individual's needs.

USING SUPPLEMENTS

When treating IBD with herbs, you might consider also using supplements. To support the work of the plants, you might try:
* Magnesium, 200 mg per day
* Multivitamin and minerals
* Vitamin A, 50,000 international units (IU) per day
* Vitamin E, 200 IU per day
* Zinc picolinate, 50 mg per day

* Astringent remedies, such as bayberry and cranesbill, are crucial in the reduction of any bleeding.
* Demulcent herbs, such as marsh mallow root, might soothe the surface irritation and can help guard against exacerbation of ulceration.
* Vulneraries will promote the healing of ulceration in the mucosal lining.
* Anti-inflammatories, such as chamomile and wild yam, will help the body get the inflammatory reaction under control.
* Carminatives, such as chamomile and lemon balm, might help ease the abdominal discomfort. Drink a warm infusion of the herb as often as needed to alleviate discomfort.
* Antispasmodics, such as cramp bark and valerian, will help ease pain caused by muscular cramping in the bowels.
* Nervines, such as chamomile and valerian, will address any stress components of this condition.

In addition, garlic has shown potential as a specific remedy for IBD; eat at least one raw clove daily as a dietary supplement.

Bayberry is an excellent astringent for use in this disease but cannot be thought of as a specific. The autoimmune basis of IBD means that you must be patient while selecting remedies, as many possible herbs can be used.

IBD Combination Tincture

From this formula you'll get anti-inflammatories (chamomile, wild yam), antispasmodics (chamomile, valerian), astringents (agrimony, bayberry, marsh mallow root), carminatives (chamomile, valerian), demulcents (marsh mallow root), and nervines (chamomile, valerian).

2 parts bayberry
2 parts marsh mallow root
2 parts wild yam
1 part agrimony
1 part chamomile
1 part valerian

To make: Mix the herbs and make a tincture following the instructions on page 113.
To use: Take up to 1 teaspoon (5 ml) three times a day.

INDIVIDUALIZING YOUR TREATMENT

The combination of herbs in IBD Combination Tincture supplies the range of actions needed to ease colon symptoms but does not directly address the immune problem. For greater astringency, increase the bayberry or agrimony. Alternatively, add cranesbill in addition to the other remedies. You might also need increased nervine activity and demulcency, but specifics will vary from person to person.

IRRITABLE BOWEL SYNDROME

Irritable bowel syndrome (IBS) is a common disorder characterized by crampy pain, gassiness, bloating, and changes in bowel habits. It might manifest as constipation or diarrhea or swing between both and can result in headaches and anxiety. Bleeding, fever, weight loss, and persistent severe pain are not symptoms of IBS and usually indicate other problems.

A whole panoply of symptoms can occur in this condition, including abdominal distress, erratic frequency of bowel movements, and variability in stool consistency. There is no "normal bowel function," as it varies from person to person — bowel movements can range from three stools a day to three a week! However, a normal movement can be described as consisting of stools that are formed but not hard, contain no blood, and pass painlessly. With IBS you might endure crampy abdominal pain with painful constipation or diarrhea, alternating constipation and diarrhea, and mucus in the stools.

IBS has very diverse and sometimes obscure causes, and while stress, anxiety, and psychological factors are often pivotal, they are but components of a larger problem. Other factors to consider include:

• Intolerance to such common foods as citrus fruits, coffee, corn, dairy products, tea, and wheat
• Intolerance to lactose
• Excessive bran consumption
• Infectious or parasitic organisms such as *Candida, Giardia,* threadworm, and many others
• Drugs, especially antibiotics

Although not the cause of IBS, a "trigger" must be present for symptoms to occur. Common triggers include diet and emotional stress.

Eating causes contractions of the colon. Normally, this induces the urge to have a bowel movement within 30 to 60 minutes.

However, in IBS this urge comes sooner and is accompanied by cramps and diarrhea. The intensity is often related to the number of calories and the amount of fat in the meal. Fat, whether animal or vegetable, is a strong stimulus of colonic contractions.

Types of IBS

The colon connects the small intestine with the rectum and anus. It's here that water and electrolytes are absorbed from material that enters from the small intestine. This material remains in the colon until most of the fluid and salts are absorbed into the body. The stool then passes through to the left side of the colon, where it is stored. Nerves, hormones, and electrical activity in the colon muscle control the contraction of intestinal muscles and movement of its contents. Movements of the colon propel the contents slowly back and forth but mainly toward the rectum. A few times a day, strong muscle contractions push fecal material ahead, often resulting in a bowel movement.

A number of factors appear to cause colitis, an inflammation of the colon. Mucous colitis, also called irritable or spastic colon, is a functional disturbance in which the colon secretes abnormally large amounts of mucus, which appears in the stools. The most common symptom is abdominal cramping accompanied by either constipation or diarrhea, sometimes alternately. Many herbs can be used to treat this condition.

Ulcerative colitis is another matter. A serious inflammatory disease that seems to be autoimmune in nature, ulcerative colitis poses real challenges to any therapist, whether herbalist or allopath. Nevertheless, a competent medical herbalist has much to offer in the treatment of this autoimmune condition.

Two extreme varieties of IBS are commonly observed, with many shades between. The "spastic colon" type is characterized by an alternation between constipation and diarrhea associated with and often triggered by eating. The other extreme is a painless but precipitous diarrhea.

The Role of Stress

It is a misconception that IBS is caused by emotional conflict or stress. Stress will definitely aggravate symptoms, but other factors are important as well. The colon of someone with IBS is more sensitive than usual, responding strongly to stimuli that would not bother most people.

Since stress stimulates colonic spasm, stress reduction training or counseling and support help relieve IBS symptoms.

Lifestyle Treatments

As with indigestion, just about anything that helps you to feel at ease or improves physiological activity is indicated for IBS. Diet is fundamental, but finding the key food triggers can be a real challenge.

Keep a journal that notes which foods seem to trigger symptoms. If dairy products cause flare-ups, eat a lot less of these foods. You might tolerate yogurt better, because it contains organisms that supply lactase, the enzyme needed to digest lactose. Large meals can cause cramping and diarrhea, so eating smaller meals more often or simply smaller portions of meals can ease symptoms. Also, meals that are low in fat and high in carbohydrates such as pasta, rice, whole-grain breads and cereals, fruits, and vegetables can help.

Dietary fiber might lessen IBS symptoms by keeping the colon mildly distended, which can help to prevent spasms. Some forms of fiber also keep water in the stools, thereby preventing hard stools that are difficult to pass. Whole-grain breads and cereals, beans, fruits, and vegetables are good sources of fiber. Eat just enough fiber so that bowel movements are painless and easily passed. A high-fiber diet might initially cause gas and bloating, but within a few weeks these symptoms subside as the body adjusts.

Treating with Herbs

Digestion and subsequent elimination are pivotal in relieving IBS, as is supporting the nervous system. Tonics can strengthen any part of the body that is a focus for energy usage and thus can enhance digestive functioning. As with indigestion, IBS is a functional problem; many general remedies are useful, but none are considered specifics.

Chamomile and peppermint are two plants that have a direct impact on an irritable bowel. With astringents such as bayberry, wound-healing remedies such as comfrey root or plantain, and the colic-relieving properties of the antispasmodic wild yam, much can be done to facilitate the healing of these distressing problems. Garlic is most valuable, but whether this is because of an antimicrobial effect or some broader action is difficult to say. Remember these general principles:

- Astringents, such as agrimony, bayberry, or meadowsweet, will reverse the diarrhea and reduce any pathological mucus production.
- Bitters, such as mugwort, will promote appropriate digestive secretions and often will normalize bowel function by themselves. Bitters also have hepatic activity that will support the liver during illness.
- Anti-inflammatories, such as chamomile, will reduce localized mucosal reaction.
- Carminatives, such as peppermint, will ease flatulence or colic. Drink a warm infusion of carminative nervines as often as needed to ease discomfort.
- Antispasmodics, such as valerian and wild yam, are indicated if the cramping is severe.
- Vulneraries are useful if your health care practitioner has diagnosed damage to the lining of the colon.
- Nervines will help ease background stress.
- Laxatives might be indicated temporarily, but do not use strong ones; the swing back to diarrhea can be quick.

Colitis Relief Tincture

This healing formula supplies anti-inflammatories (chamomile, wild yam), antispasmodics (chamomile, peppermint, wild yam), astringents (bayberry), bitters (mugwort, chamomile), carminatives (chamomile, peppermint), nervines (chamomile, valerian), and vulneraries (chamomile). An infusion of a carminative, such as peppermint, will support the work of the tincture.

2 parts bayberry	1 part peppermint
1 part chamomile	1 part valerian
1 part mugwort	1 part wild yam

To make: Mix the herbs and make a tincture following the instructions on page 113.

To use: Take up to 1 teaspoon (5 ml) three times a day.

PEPTIC ULCERATION

Ulcerative conditions of the stomach, duodenum, and esophagus are very common in our society, and nonprescription medicines for these conditions are major moneymakers for the pharmaceutical industry. Drug treatment is based primarily upon reducing the corrosive impact of stomach acid on the mucosal lining. This is done through antacid chemicals or other agents that reduce acid production, either directly or indirectly. But a range of plants are available that appear to work in a broader way to help reverse the syndrome.

The Different Types of Ulceration

Peptic ulcers usually have a chronic, recurrent course, with variable symptoms. In fact, only about half of all ulcer patients have the "characteristic" picture, describing the pain as burning, gnawing, or aching and the distress as a soreness, empty feeling, or "hunger." Antacids or milk relieve the pain. The main cause of peptic ulcer is bacterial infection, but long-term use of non-steroidal anti-inflammatory agents (NSAIDs), such as aspirin and ibuprofen, can cause ulcers as well. Occasionally, cancerous tumors in the stomach or pancreas cause ulcers.

Duodenal ulcers, on the other hand, are typically described as feeling like hunger pains. They are usually relieved by eating. These ulcers can be caused by a range of factors, including bacterial infection, stress, drug therapy (especially with NSAIDs), exposure to chemical irritants (such as alcohol, coffee, and tobacco), and even your own genetic makeup.

Gastric ulcers have generally the same causes as duodenal ulcers. Gastric ulcers can be brought on by eating, and symptoms include abdominal pain, nausea, vomiting, and even weight loss and fatigue.

Problems to Avoid

There are some common consequences of the nonherbal treatment of peptic ulceration:

- Excessive use of antacids can lead to the impaired absorption of certain nutrients from the diet.
- Milk consumption might aggravate problems associated with a sensitivity to dairy products.
- Eating a bland, milky, carbohydrate-rich diet might lead to obesity.
- Excessive drinking of milk or consumption of antacids can lead to elevated levels of calcium in body tissues and urine, which might lead to kidney stones.
- A poor appetite associated with ulceration might lead to nutritional deficit.

Lifestyle Treatments

Dietary factors are fundamentally involved in both the cause and treatment of peptic ulceration. In some cases, a specific food allergy might have caused the ulceration, but sensitivity to irritants will continue to aggravate the ulcer. As in the other digestive system conditions discussed here, it's imperative to avoid all such irritant foods — especially alcohol and tobacco. Remove from your diet pepper, coffee, and anything that causes your symptoms. Small meals often are better than large meals. Increasing the proportion of fiber in the diet has been shown to reduce the rate of recurrence of peptic ulceration; however, the early stages of treatment should include a bland diet to avoid physical irritation.

Other essential steps to take are to rest, avoid aspirin and other nonsteroidal anti-inflammatories, and reevaluate a lifestyle that might be causing stress. Make it a priority to create a stress management program uniquely suited for your needs.

Treating with Herbs

With the skilled use of herbs it is very possible to rapidly and completely heal a peptic ulcer. The actions most indicated for ulceration include:

- Demulcents, which protectively coat and soothe the lining of the stomach
- Anti-inflammatories, which reduce the local mucosal reaction
- Astringents, which lessen any bleeding
- Vulneraries, which speed up natural wound healing
- Carminatives, which ease any subsequent flatulence lower down in the abdomen
- Nervines, which help ease stress

Herbs such as calendula, chamomile, comfrey root, goldenseal, marsh mallow root, and meadowsweet are examples of the remedies that can be used for peptic ulceration. Drink an infusion of the fresh or dried herbs often to ease symptoms. Drinking chamomile infusion on an empty stomach will reduce inflammation and help reverse the ulcerative process.

Inflammation Reducer

Treating peptic ulceration with herbs is a two-stage process. The first, which you'll find in this recipe, reduces inflammation and initiates healing through demulcents and vulneraries. You can also drink infusions of the fresh or dried herbs often to ease symptoms. See the recipe on page 71 for the second step.

1 part chamomile
1 part comfrey root
1 part marsh mallow root

To make: Mix the herbs and make a tincture following the instructions on page 113.
To use: Take 1 teaspoon (5 ml) three times a day until symptoms are alleviated.

WHEN TO SEEK EMERGENCY CARE

If you experience any of the following symptoms, seek professional help immediately.
• Sharp, sudden, persistent stomach pain
• Bloody or black stools
• Bloody vomit or vomit that looks like coffee grounds

Ulcer Healing Formula

After using the above formula for the appropriate amount of time, tone and complete healing with this remedy. From these formulas, you'll get anti-inflammatories (chamomile, goldenseal), astringents (comfrey root, goldenseal), bitters (goldenseal), carminatives (chamomile), demulcents (comfrey root, marsh mallow root), nervines (chamomile), and vulneraries (chamomile, comfrey root, goldenseal).

Note: *If symptoms have not subsided within a week, seek the assistance of a health care professional.*

> 2 parts chamomile
> 2 parts comfrey root
> 1 part goldenseal

To make: Mix the herbs and make a tincture following the instructions on page 113.
To use: Take 1 teaspoon (5ml) three times a day.

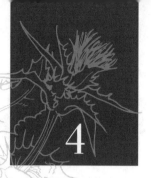

TREATING
COMMON LIVER DISEASES

L iver disease is an area of therapy well suited to herbal treatment. Whether the condition requires gentle liver stimulation or profound disease treatment, we have a robust materia medica from which we can draw remedies. Pharmacological and clinical research is starting to support the traditional experience of the medical herbalist and provide chemical insight into the mechanisms involved.

On the other hand, conventional medicine does not provide many remedies for hepatitis, cirrhosis, liver damage caused by toxins, or biliary tract disorders. Patients with liver disorders are usually given supportive treatment (modified diet; removal of toxins such as drugs or alcohol) rather than active therapy. Both Western and Chinese systems have long utilized herbs for such problems.

FUNCTIONS OF THE LIVER

The liver is the largest solid organ in the body, with a wide range of functions. These include:

- Metabolism of protein
- Initiation of the formation of bile
- Metabolism of carbohydrates as well as the storage of glycogen
- Metabolism of lipids, including the synthesis of cholesterol and bile acids
- Biotransformation (chemical changing) of waste, toxins, and drugs so that they can be removed from the bloodstream via the kidneys
- Production of blood-clotting factors and other blood proteins

In addition, reticulo-endothelial cells (the Kupffer cells), which are part of the liver, play a role in immunity. The liver is able to regenerate itself after injury or disease. If, however, a disease progresses beyond the tissue's capacity to generate new cells, the body's entire metabolism is severely affected. Any number of disorders can affect the liver and interfere with the blood supply, the hepatic and Kupffer cells, and the bile ducts.

What Causes Liver Disease?

The main causes of liver disease are viral infection and hepatotoxic chemicals (chemicals that are toxic to the liver) such as ethyl alcohol, peroxides (particularly peroxidized cooking oil), pollutants and synthetic chemicals in food, pharmaceuticals, and environmental pollutants. Although such liver lesions induced by these toxins can be reversed in the early stages, they can be healed only by removal of the toxins.

Taking an Herbal Approach

In the face of the many toxic challenges presented by modern life, the green world can offer some help. A number of herbs long used for liver disorders, especially milk thistle, have revealed their unique potential under pharmacological investigation. Anti-

hepatotoxicity appears to be due to a combination of two main mechanisms:
- An alteration of cell membranes, such that only small amounts of toxins may penetrate into the cell, and
- An acceleration of protein synthesis, thus stimulating cell regeneration.

JAUNDICE

Jaundice, or yellowing of the skin and the whites of the eyes, is a symptom and not a disease in itself. Jaundice can be caused by disease of the liver cells, obstruction of the bile ducts, or immaturity of the liver (as in newborns); besides discoloration of the skin, other symptoms associated with jaundice can include intense

Jaundice Tincture

This formula supplies the range of actions needed to relieve jaundice, including alteratives and tonics (dandelion root), antihepatotoxics (milk thistle), antipruritics (chickweed), bitters (dandelion root, vervain), and hepatics (dandelion root, milk thistle, vervain).

2 parts dandelion root
1 part milk thistle
1 part vervain

To make: Mix the herbs and make a tincture following the instructions on page 113.
To use: Take up to ½ teaspoon (2.5 ml) three times a day, increasing, over a period of a week, to 1 teaspoon (5 ml) three times a day. Continue taking the tincture for two weeks following the alleviation of symptoms.

itching and general malaise. Careful diagnosis is required to determine the cause and treatment needed.

The most common cause of jaundice is cholestasis, a disease stemming from a variety of processes, in which the flow of bile is impaired. This blockage causes a backup of bilirubin, the pigment produced when the liver processes waste products, which in turn leads to jaundice. The cause of the blockage must be determined; it can be inflamed tissues, ducts blocked by gallstones, cancer, or even parasites.

Treating with Herbs

In Europe, dandelion root and vervain have traditionally been considered specific remedies for jaundice. To prevent hepatotoxicity from backed-up bile, employ the liver cell–regenerative potentials of milk thistle. In addition:

- Cholagogue remedies, such as dandelion root and vervain, directly stimulate secretion and release of bile.
- Hepatics can improve metabolic functioning of the liver.
- Bitters, such as boldo and the cholagogues, act as tonics and often support metabolic functioning.
- Antihepatotoxic support, such as that from milk thistle, is essential to minimize liver damage from any bile buildup.
- Alteratives and tonics will support the body as a whole in its healing work.
- Antipruritics (agents that reduce itching) are helpful in some cases. Apply an infusion of chickweed or distilled witch hazel to relieve discomfort.

HEPATITIS

This serious disease can be due to a range of causes, including:

- Viral infection, which is often extremely contagious

- Bacteria or other microorganisms
- Parasitic infestation
- Toxic damage due to alcohol or other drugs (both recreational and therapeutic), as well as some plant poisons such as pyrolizadine alkaloids

Diagnosing whether the problem is viral hepatitis, chronic nonviral hepatitis, or alcohol-induced liver disease is crucial. However, all forms of active hepatitis are characterized by malaise, anorexia, and fatigue; they are sometimes initiated with flulike symptoms and often are associated with a range of specific signs, from vomiting to jaundice. The information given here is of most relevance to hepatitis A and B, and, to a lesser extent, hepatitis C.

Treating with Herbs

There is potentially a whole constellation of pathologies present in hepatitis, so finding specific herbs is problematic. Milk thistle's hepato-regenerative potential makes this plant the closest to a textbook specific remedy. All the tonic hepatics are relevant and include balmony, dandelion root, and fringetree bark. Also, remember that:

- Hepatics have a positive effect upon liver metabolism and functioning.
- Antimicrobials will be crucial if there is an infection present. Even if the herbs cannot treat the specific virus, they will provide immune support.
- Bitters contribute their unique brand of whole body toning.
- Cholagogues are remedies that directly affect the secretion and release of bile; they might be indicated if jaundice is present.
- Antihepatotoxic support is essential to minimize liver damage from any bile buildup.
- Alteratives and tonics will support the body as a whole in its healing work.

Keep in mind that some forms of hepatitis can be fatal. Regardless of what type of hepatitis you are treating or what kinds of herbs you would like to try, you *must* seek the diagnosis and supervision of a physician and herbalist.

Milk Thistle Hepatitis Remedy

A gentle, non-irritating combination of herbs, this remedy facilitates regeneration of damaged liver cells.

2 parts milk thistle   1 part echinacea
1 part dandelion root   1 part fringetree bark

To make: Mix the herbs and make a tincture following the instructions on page 113.
To use: Take up to ½ teaspoon (2.5 ml) three times a day, increasing over a one week period to 1 teaspoon (5 ml) three times a day.

CHOLECYSTITIS (GALLBLADDER INFLAMMATION)

The gallbladder is a small pear-shaped organ located beneath the liver on the right side of the abdomen. Its primary functions are to store and concentrate bile, secreting it into the small intestine at the proper time to help digest food. The gallbladder is connected to the liver and the small intestine by a series of ducts, or tube-shaped structures. Collectively, the gallbladder and these ducts are called the biliary system.

The liver produces bile, a yellow-brown fluid containing water, cholesterol, fats, bile salts, and bilirubin, the pigment that gives stools their color. The liver can produce as much as three cups of bile in one day, and the gallbladder can store up to a cup of concentrated bile.

Cholecystitis, or gallbladder inflammation, is characterized by severe pain localized in the upper right quadrant of the abdomen radiating to the right lower scapula (the shoulder bone that is connected to the collarbone). Nausea and vomiting are common. Murphy's sign — a sensitivity experienced when the area just under the right ribs is pressed — is found. Given time, cholecystitis responds well to herbal treatment, but the affected person might resist treatment due to the extreme pain the condition produces. Paying attention to diet is pivotal; any fats will intensify the pain.

Allopathic medicine tends to downplay the role of the gallbladder and of bile in digestion. That might be why the gallbladder is so often surgically removed when gallstones are present. People are said to lead perfectly normal lives after gallbladder removal, but the presence of a healthy gallbladder helps ensure effective digestion and thus directly decreases the chances of arteriosclerosis, irritable bowel syndrome, hypertension, heart disease, stroke, and other diseases.

Treating with Herbs

Several types of herbs are valuable for treating cholecystitis: *Caution:* Bitters and strong cholagogues are contraindicated because they increase the strength of muscle contraction.

- Hepatic tonics will support the work of the liver and therefore have a positive metabolic effect.
- Anti-inflammatories help reduce the severity of swelling.
- Antihepatotoxic support is essential to minimize liver damage from any bile buildup.
- Nervines help ease the strain from pain and general worry.
- Antispasmodics might help ease the colic in the gallbladder or gallbladder ducts.

In addition, take an infusion of an herb with antispasmodic, carminative, and nervine action regularly throughout the day. Chamomile is an excellent example.

Gallbladder Soother

This formula supplies antilithic (stone-preventing), antispasmodic, hepatic, and nervine actions. Many herbalists also recommend balmony, goldenseal (in small amounts), lobelia, Oregon grape, and vervain as part of their mixtures. In addition, you can use an infusion of an antispasmodic, carminative, nervine herb (such as chamomile) in conjunction with the tincture.

2 parts fringetree bark	1 part black root
2 parts valerian	1 part dandelion root
2 parts wild yam	

To make: Mix the herbs and make a tincture following the instructions on page 113.
To use: Take up to 1 teaspoon (5 ml) three times a day.

GALLSTONES

Gallstones are solid materials that form in the gallbladder when substances in the bile — primarily cholesterol and bile pigments — form hard, crystal-like particles. The stones can vary in size from as small as a grain of sand to as large as a golf ball. The gallbladder can develop a single, often large, stone or a variety of smaller ones.

Gallstones appear to be caused by a combination of factors, including a person's inherited body chemistry, body weight, gallbladder activity, and diet. It has been estimated that 20 million

Americans have gallstones. Those who are most likely to develop them are:

- Women between 20 and 60 years of age.
- Men and women over 60.
- Pregnant women or women who have used birth control pills or estrogen replacement therapy.
- Native Americans. This group has the highest prevalence of gallstones in the United States. A majority of Native American men have gallstones by age 60.
- Men and women who are overweight.
- People who go on crash diets or lose a lot of weight quickly.

Most people who have gallstones have no symptoms; a doctor detects the stones during a routine medical checkup or examination for another illness. But for some people the stones can be excruciatingly painful. This pain is a steady, severe pain in the upper abdomen but can also be present in the back between the shoulder blades or in the right shoulder. Nausea or vomiting can result. Attacks can be separated by weeks, months, or even years.

The exclusion of fats from the diet is essential in relieving gallstones. Attention to stress reduction is also important. Pharmaceutical pain relievers will be indicated in the severe cases.

Treating with Herbs

Take an infusion of a carminative, antispasmodic, nervine herb, such as chamomile, regularly throughout the day. *Caution:* Bitters and strong cholagogues are contraindicated, because they increase the strength of muscle contraction. You'll find several other herbs helpful for gallstones:

- Antilithic plants have a long tradition of use in easing the pain, movement, and even dissolving of gallstones. They include balmony, black root, and fringetree bark.
- Nervines help ease the strain from pain and general worry.

- Although their mechanism of action is not completely understood, hepatic tonics will support the work of the liver.
- Antispasmodics might help ease the colic in the gallbladder or gallbladder ducts.
- Antihepatotoxic support is essential to minimize liver damage from any bile buildup.

Gallstone Remedy

You can also use an infusion of a carminative, antispasmodic, nervine herb in conjunction with this tincture. Given time, the tincture will improve the condition itself, but it will not ease the extreme pain associated with gallstones.

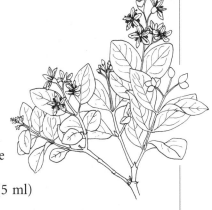

2 parts boldo
2 parts valerian
2 parts wild yam
1 part balmony
1 part black root
1 part fringetree bark

To make: Mix the herbs and make a tincture following the instructions on page 113.
To use: Take up to 1 teaspoon (5 ml) three times a day.

A DIRECTORY OF HERBS
FOR HEALTHY DIGESTION

Herbs have been used for centuries to treat a wide variety of ailments. Although herbs have been largely disregarded by allopathic medicine, researchers are now rediscovering what herbalists have known all along: Phytotherapy, or treatment with plants, affords us more versatility with far less adverse reactions than do chemical drugs.

The green world offers us a veritable cornucopia of healing herbs. Careful selection from this rich abundance can provide a range of safe, effective, and pleasant healing agents for both maintaining the health of the digestive system and treating many of its maladies. The herbs described in this section are those most likely to be of help for the various conditions described in this book. These herbs have been selected for their efficacy, ease of use, and availability.

AGRIMONY *(Agrimonia eupatoria)*

Parts Used: Aerial parts
Actions: Antispasmodic, astringent, bitter, carminative, cholagogue, diuretic, hepatic, tonic, vulnerary
Indications: Agrimony is indicated when an astringent action on the digestive system is needed. It is used as a treatment for diarrhea

and especially in the treatment of irritable bowel syndrome and colitis. This plant can also be useful in urinary incontinence and cystitis. As a gargle it eases the discomfort of sore throats and laryngitis. As an ointment it aids the healing of wounds and bruises.

Preparations and Dosage: Make an infusion by pouring 1 cup boiling water over 1–2 teaspoons of the dried herb and steep for 10–15 minutes. Drink one cup three times a day.

As a tincture, take 1–4 ml three times a day.

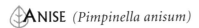 ANISE *(Pimpinella anisum)*

Part Used: Seeds

Actions: Antimicrobial, antispasmodic, aromatic, carminative, expectorant, galactogogue

Indications: The volatile oil in aniseed provides the basis for its internal use to ease griping, intestinal colic, and flatulence. It also has antispasmodic and expectorant actions; use it for bronchitis, for tracheitis in which there is persistent irritable coughing, and for whooping cough. Use the oil externally in an ointment base for the treatment of scabies. The oil by itself will control lice. Anise has mild estrogenic effects, thought to be due to the presence of volatile oils known to be phytoestrogens, which explains the use of this plant in folk medicine to increase milk secretion, facilitate birth, and increase libido.

Combinations: For flatulent colic, mix aniseed with equal amounts of caraway and fennel. For bronchitis, combine with coltsfoot, horehound, and lobelia.

Preparations and Dosage: Make an infusion by gently crushing the seeds. Pour 1 cup boiling water over 1–2 teaspoons of the seeds and let stand, covered, for 5–10 minutes. Take one cup three times daily. For flatulence, drink the tea slowly before meals.

One drop of food-grade aniseed essential oil mixed with ½ teaspoon honey can be taken internally before meals, but only under the supervision of a qualified herbalist.

BALMONY *(Chelone glabra)*

Parts Used: Dried aerial parts

Actions: Antiemetic (nausea preventive or reliever), cholagogue, hepatic, laxative, stimulant

Indications: Balmony, also called turtlehead, is an excellent remedy for liver problems. It acts as a tonic on the whole digestive system. It also has a stimulating effect on the secretion of digestive juices, making it a laxative as well. Balmony is used to treat cholecystitis, gallstones, and jaundice and is considered a specific for gallstones that lead to congestive jaundice. It stimulates the appetite, eases colic, dyspepsia, and biliousness and is helpful for weakness. Externally it has been used on inflamed breast tissue, painful ulcers, and piles.

Combinations: For relief of constipation, combine balmony with butternut. For jaundice, combine it with milk thistle and other toning hepatics such as goldenseal.

Preparations and Dosage: To make an infusion, pour 1 cup boiling water over 2 teaspoons of the dried herb and steep for 10–15 minutes. Drink one cup three times a day.

As a tincture, take 1–2 ml three times a day.

BARBERRY *(Berberis spp.)*

Parts Used: Bark of the root or stem

Actions: Antiemetic, bitter, cholagogue, hepatic, laxative

Indications: Barberry is one of the best remedies for correcting liver function and promoting the flow of bile. It is indicated when there are gallstones or inflammation of the gallbladder or when jaundice occurs due to a congested state of the liver. As a bitter tonic with mild laxative effects, it is used in debilitated people to strengthen and cleanse the system. This herb also has the ability to reduce an enlarged spleen. It acts against malaria and is also effective in the treatment of protozoal infection due to *Leishmania* spp. *Caution:* Avoid barberry during pregnancy.

Combinations: For gallbladder diseases, combine barberry with fringetree bark and black root.

Preparations and Dosage: To make a decoction, add 1 teaspoon of the bark to 1 cup cold water and bring to a boil. Remove from heat and steep for 10–15 minutes. Drink one cup of tea three times a day.

As a tincture, take 1–2 ml three times a day.

BLACK HAW *(Viburnum prunifolium)*

Parts Used: Dried bark of root, stem, or trunk

Actions: Antispasmodic, astringent, hypotensive, nervine

Indications: Black haw is used similarly to cramp bark, a close relative. It is a powerful relaxant of the uterus and is used for dysmenorrhea (painful menstruation), false labor pains, and in threatened miscarriage. Its relaxant and sedative actions make it a powerful blood pressure reducer, and thus it is often used to treat hypertension. It is also used as an antispasmodic in the treatment of asthma.

Preparations and Dosage: To make a decoction, add 2 teaspoons of the dried bark to 1 cup cold water. Bring to a boil and simmer for 10 minutes. Drink one cup three times a day.

As a tincture, take 5–10 ml three times a day.

BLACK ROOT *(Veronicastrum virginicum)*

Parts Used: Rhizome and root

Actions: Antispasmodic, cholagogue, diaphoretic, hepatic, laxative

Indications: Also known as Culver's root, black root relieves liver congestion and inflammation of the gallbladder (cholecystitis). Use black root when jaundice is due to liver congestion. This herb is also ideal when liver dysfunction leads to chronic constipation.

Combinations: Black root combines well with barberry and dandelion root to stimulate bile flow. For hemorrhoids, combine with stone root.

Preparations and Dosage: To make a decoction, add 1–2 teaspoons of the dried herb to 1 cup cold water and bring to a boil. Simmer for 10 minutes. Strain, and drink one cup three times a day.

As a tincture, take 1–2 ml three times a day.

BOLDO *(Peumus boldo)*

Part Used: Dried leaves

Actions: Cholagogue, diuretic, hepatic

Indications: Boldo is a specific for gallbladder problems such as stones or inflammation. It is also used when there is visceral pain due to other problems in the liver or gallbladder. Boldo has mild urinary demulcent and antiseptic properties and is used in cystitis.

Combinations: When treating gallbladder or liver problems, combine with fringetree bark and mountain grape.

Preparations and Dosage: To make an infusion, pour 1 cup boiling water over 1 teaspoon of the dried leaves and steep 10–15 minutes. Drink one cup three times a day.

As a tincture, take 1–2 ml three times a day.

BONESET *(Eupatorium perfoliatum)*

Parts Used: Dried aerial parts

Actions: Antispasmodic, astringent, bitter, carminative, diaphoretic, laxative, tonic

Indications: Boneset is one of the best remedies for the relief of the symptoms that accompany influenza. It speedily relieves the aches and pains as well as helping the body deal with fever. Boneset can also be used to help clear the upper respiratory tract of mucous congestion. Its mild laxative activity will ease constipation. It can safely be used as a general cleansing agent. Boneset is also used in the treatment of muscle pain or muscular rheumatism.

Combinations: In the treatment of influenza, combine boneset with cayenne, elder flowers, ginger, or yarrow. Mix with elecampane and pleurisy root for bronchial conditions.

Preparations and Dosage: To make an infusion, pour 1 cup boiling water over 1–2 teaspoons of the dried herb and steep for 10–15 minutes. Drink the liquid as hot as possible every half hour when treating fevers or flus.

As a tincture, take 2–4 ml three times a day.

BUTTERNUT *(Juglans cinerea)*

Part Used: Inner bark

Actions: Anthelmintic (destroys parasites), cholagogue, laxative

Indications: Butternut is used as an antihemorrhoidal, cholagogue, dermatological agent, and laxative. Finley Ellingwood, in *American Materia Medica,* says, "Experiments with the [herb] have ascertained that it influences, with great energy, the liver, small intestines, colon and rectum, causing an increased manufacture and elimination of bile, as well as increased activity of the glands of the intestinal tract. Full doses produce large bilious evacuations, without much pain or griping." He suggests the use of butternut in acne, chronic jaundice, constipation, eczema, herpes, impetigo, and pemphigus.

Preparation and Dosage: As a tincture, take 1–2 ml at night and in the morning.

CELERY SEED *(Apium graveolens)*

Part Used: Dried ripe seeds

Actions: Anti-inflammatory, antirheumatic (alleviates rheumatism), antispasmodic, carminative, diuretic, nervine

Indications: Celery seeds are mainly used in the treatment of arthritis, gout, and rheumatism. They are especially useful in rheumatoid arthritis where there is an associated mental depression. Celery seeds' diuretic action is obviously involved in rheumatic conditions, but it is also used as a urinary antiseptic — largely because of the volatile oil apiol.

Combinations: In rheumatic conditions, celery seed combines well with bogbean.

Preparations and Dosage: To make an infusion, pour 1 cup boiling water over 1–2 teaspoons of freshly crushed seeds. Steep for 10–15 minutes. Drink one cup three times a day.

As a tincture, take 1–4 ml three times a day.

CHAMOMILE, GERMAN (*Matricaria recutita*) AND ROMAN (*Chamaemelum nobile*)

Part Used: Flowers

Actions: Anti-inflammatory, antimicrobial, antispasmodic, bitter, carminative, nervine, vulnerary

Indications: A comprehensive list of chamomile's medical uses would be very long. It might seem too good to be true, but chamomile is used for a wide range of ailments, including aches and pains of flu, anxiety, colic, conjunctivitis, diarrhea, dyspepsia, inflamed skin, insomnia, loss of appetite, menopausal depression, migraine, motion sickness, neuralgia, teething, urticaria (hives), and vertigo.

Chamomile is probably the most widely used relaxing nervine herb in the Western world. It relaxes and tones the nervous system and is especially valuable where anxiety and tension produce digestive symptoms such as colic pains, gas, or even ulcers. Being rich in essential oil, it promotes proper function of the digestive system. This usually involves soothing the walls of the intestines, easing griping pains, and helping in the removal of gas. A cup of hot chamomile tea is a simple, effective way to relieve indigestion, calm inflammations such as gastritis, and help prevent ulcer formation. Safe in all types of stress and anxiety related problems, chamomile makes a wonderful late night tea to ensure restful sleep.

As an antispasmodic herb, chamomile works on the peripheral nerves and muscles and thus indirectly relaxes the whole body. When the physical body is at ease, ease in the mind and heart follow. Chamomile can prevent or ease cramps in the muscles, such as in the legs or abdomen. The essential oil added to a bath relaxes the body after a hard day while easing the cares of a troubled heart and mind.

This popular herb is also an effective anti-inflammatory remedy for the respiratory system and externally, on the skin. Use the essential oil as a steam inhalation to ease inflamed mucous membranes in the sinuses and lungs. As an anticatarrhal it helps the body remove excess mucus buildup in the sinus area. Use it to treat head colds and allergy reactions such as hay fever. Add chamomile to the bath to soothe anxious children or teething infants.

Chamomile is a mild antimicrobial, helping the body to destroy or resist pathogenic microorganisms. Azulene, one of the components of the essential oil, is bactericidal to *Staphylococcus* and *Streptococcus* infections. The oil from .10 grams of flowers is enough to destroy three times that amount of staphylococcal toxins in two hours' time!

VERSATILE CHAMOMILE

A review of recent scientific literature shows how much interest this venerable folk remedy is still receiving. Most of the clinical, therapeutic research comes from Europe, where the anti-inflammatory effects have been the main focus of research on chamomile. This action is the official criteria for chamomile's inclusion in the *German Pharmacopoeia*.

Taken by mouth or used as an enema, chamomile is particularly helpful in colitis and irritable bowel syndrome. A fascinating German study demonstrated chamomile's effectiveness in healing the wounds caused by tattooing, where it decreases the weeping of the wound and dramatically speeds drying.

Preparations and Dosage: The plant can be used in all types of medicinal preparations; the essential oil is particularly valued in aromatherapy. Do not use the essential oil during pregnancy unless instructed by an herbalist.

To make an infusion, pour 1 cup boiling water over 2–3 teaspoons fresh or 1 teaspoon dried herb. Steep for 10 minutes. Drink one cup three to four times a day.

The tincture is an excellent way of ensuring that all the plant's components are extracted and available for the body. Take 1–4 ml three times a day.

CRAMP BARK *(Viburnum opulus)*

Part Used: Dried bark
Actions: Anti-inflammatory, antispasmodic, astringent, emmenagogue, hypotensive, nervine
Indications: Cramp bark's name displays its richly deserved reputation as a relaxer of muscular tension and spasm. The herb, which is commonly called European cranberry bush, is often used to relax the uterus and relieve painful cramps associated with menstruation (dysmenorrhea). It can also be used to protect against miscarriage. Cramp bark's astringent action gives it a role in the treatment of excessive blood loss in periods and bleeding associated with menopause. Purchase cramp bark in an herb store, rather than trying to wildcraft (harvest from the wild) it yourself.
Preparations and Dosage: To make a decoction, add 2 teaspoons of the dried bark to 1 cup cold water and bring to a boil. Simmer gently for 10–15 minutes. Strain, and drink one cup of hot tea three times a day.

As a tincture, take 4–8 ml three times a day.

CRANESBILL *(Geranium maculatum)*

Part Used: Rhizome
Actions: Antihemorrhagic (stops hemorrhaging), anti-inflammatory, astringent, vulnerary
Indications: American cranesbill is an effective astringent used to treat diarrhea, dysentery, and hemorrhoids. When bleeding accompanies duodenal or gastric ulceration, this remedy is used in

combination with other relevant herbs. Cranesbill can also be used in cases of blood loss through the feces, though careful diagnosis is vital. It will help stop excessive blood loss during menstruation (menorrhagia) or a uterine hemorrhage (metrorrhagia). Use as a douche for leukorrhea (white or yellowish viscid vaginal discharge).

Preparations and Dosage: To make a decoction, add 1–2 teaspoons of the chopped rhizome to 1 cup cold water and bring to a boil. Simmer for 10–15 minutes. Drink one cup three times a day.

As a tincture, take 2–4 ml three times a day.

DANDELION *(Taraxacum officinale)*

Parts Used: Root or leaf

Actions: Antirheumatic, bitter, cholagogue, diuretic, hepatic, laxative, tonic

Indications: Dandelion leaf is a very powerful diuretic and one of the best natural sources of potassium. Thus, it makes an ideally balanced diuretic that can be used safely wherever such an action is needed, including in cases of water retention due to heart problems. Use dandelion root as a hepatic and cholagogue for inflammation and congestion of the liver and gallbladder. It is specific for cases of congestive jaundice. For muscular rheumatism, dandelion is most effective as part of a wider treatment. This herb is a valuable general tonic and perhaps the best widely applicable diuretic and liver tonic.

Combinations: For liver and gallbladder problems, combine with balmony or barberry. For water retention, use with couch grass or even yarrow.

Preparations and Dosage: To make a decoction, add 2–3 teaspoons of the root to 1 cup cold water. Bring to boil and gently simmer for 10–15 minutes. Drink one cup three times a day. Eat the leaves raw in salads.

As a tincture, take 5–10 ml three times a day.

DILL *(Anethum graveolens)*

Part Used: Seeds

Actions: Anti-inflammatory, antispasmodic, aromatic, carminative, galactogogue

Indications: Dill is an excellent remedy for flatulence and the colic sometimes associated with excess gas. This is the herb of choice for colic in children. It also stimulates the flow of milk in nursing mothers. Chewing dill seeds helps clear bad breath.

Preparations and Dosage: To make an infusion, pour 1 cup boiling water over 1–2 teaspoons of gently crushed seeds. Steep for 10–15 minutes. To treat flatulence, drink one cup before meals.

As a tincture, take 1–2 ml three times a day.

FENNEL *(Foeniculum vulgare)*

Part Used: Seeds

Actions: Anti-inflammatory, antispasmodic, aromatic, carminative, galactogogue, hepatic

Indications: Fennel is an excellent stomach and intestinal remedy; it relieves flatulence and colic while stimulating digestion and appetite. It is similar to aniseed in its calming effect on bronchitis and coughs and can be used to flavor cough remedies. Fennel also increases the flow of milk in nursing mothers.

Preparations and Dosage: To make an infusion, pour 1 cup boiling water over 1–2 teaspoons of slightly crushed seeds. Steep for 10 minutes. Drink one cup three times a day. To ease flatulence, drink one cup a half hour before meals.

As a tincture, take 1–2 ml three times a day.

FRINGETREE BARK *(Chionanthus virginicus)*

Part Used: Bark of root

Actions: Alterative, antiemetic, cholagogue, diuretic, hepatic, laxative, tonic

Indications: This valuable herb is safely used for all liver problems, especially when they have developed into jaundice. It is a specific for the treatment of gallbladder inflammation and a valuable part of treating gallstones. Fringetree bark aids the liver in general and therefore is often used as part of a wider treatment for the whole body. Through its bile-releasing action it acts as a gentle and effective laxative.

Combinations: For the treatment of liver and gallbladder conditions, combine with barberry, wahoo, or wild yam.

Preparations and Dosage: To make an infusion, pour 1 cup boiling water over 1–2 teaspoons of the bark. Steep for 10–15 minutes. Drink one cup three times a day.

As a tincture, take 1–2 ml three times a day.

GARLIC *(Allium sativum)*

Part Used: Bulb

Actions: Antimicrobial, antispasmodic, cholagogue, diaphoretic, hypotensive

Indications: Garlic is among the few herbs that have a universal usage and recognition. Its daily usage aids and supports the body in ways that no other herb does. It is one of the most effective antimicrobial plants available, acting on alimentary parasites, bacteria, and viruses. The volatile oil is an effective agent and is used in infections such as chronic bronchitis, respiratory catarrh, and recurrent colds and influenza. It can be helpful in the treatment of whooping cough and as part of a broader approach to bronchitic asthma. In general garlic can be used as a preventive for most infectious conditions, digestive as well as respiratory. In the digestive tract garlic supports the development of the natural bacterial flora while killing pathogenic organisms.

In addition to these amazing properties, garlic has an international reputation for lowering both blood pressure and blood cholesterol levels and generally improving the health of the cardiovascular system. Garlic should be thought of as a daily-use basic food that will augment the body's health. It has been used externally for the treatment of ringworm and threadworm.

Preparations and Dosage: Eat one clove three times a day. If the odor becomes a problem, take three garlic oil capsules a day as a prophylactic, or take three capsules three times a day when a respiratory infection occurs.

GARLIC AND CHOLESTEROL REDUCTION

In a recent study, two groups — one consisting of 20 healthy volunteers and the other of 62 patients with coronary heart disease and raised serum cholesterol — were fed garlic for six months. All patients showed lowered cholesterol rates; the improvements reached a peak at the end of eight months. The improvement in cholesterol levels persisted throughout the two months of clinical follow-up. The clinicians concluded that garlic's essential oil possessed a distinct hypolipidemic, or fat-reducing, action in both healthy people and patients with coronary heart disease.

GENTIAN *(Gentiana lutea, G. andrewsii)*

Parts Used: Dried rhizome and root

Actions: Anthelmintic, bitter, cholagogue, emmenagogue, hepatic, sialagogue (saliva promoter)

Indications: Gentian, or yellow gentian, is an excellent bitter that encourages appetite and digestion by stimulating digestive juices and increasing the production of saliva, gastric juices, and bile. It also accelerates the emptying of the stomach. It is indicated wherever there is a lack of appetite, dyspepsia, or flatulence. Bitters' general toning effects give this herb a role in treating anorexia, debility, and exhaustion.

Preparations and Dosage: To make a decoction, add ½ teaspoon of the shredded root to 1 cup water and boil for 5 minutes. Drink warm 15–30 minutes before meals or at any time stomach pains result from a feeling of fullness.

As a tincture, take 1–2 ml three times a day.

GINGER *(Zingiber officinale)*

Part Used: Rootstock

Actions: Antispasmodic, carminative, diaphoretic, emmenagogue, rubefacient (increases blood flow to the skin), stimulant

Indications: Ginger is used as a stimulant of peripheral circulation in cases of bad circulation, chilblains, and cramps. In feverish conditions, ginger is a useful diaphoretic, promoting perspiration. It is an effective gargle for sore throats. Externally, the herb is the base of many fibrositis (tissue disorder) and muscle sprain treatments. Ginger is used worldwide as an aromatic carminative and pungent appetite stimulant. In India and other countries with hot and humid climates, ginger is eaten daily and is a well-known remedy for digestive problems. Its widespread use is credited to its flavor, as well as its antimicrobial and antioxidant effects, which are necessary for preservation of food in hot climates.

Preparations and Dosage: To make an infusion, pour 1 cup boiling water over 1 teaspoon of the fresh root and let infuse for 5 minutes. Drink whenever needed to stimulate circulation and generally warm the system.

To make a decoction, add 1½ teaspoons of the dried root (in powdered or finely chopped form) to 1 cup water. Bring to a boil and simmer for 5–10 minutes. Drink whenever needed to relieve colic pain or discomfort.

The tincture comes in two forms: weak Tincture B.P., which should be taken in a dose of 1.5–3 ml three times a day; and strong Tincture B.P., which should be taken in a dose of 0.25–0.5 ml three times a day.

GOLDENSEAL *(Hydrastis canadensis)*

Parts Used: Root and rhizome

Actions: Alterative, anticatarrhal, anti-inflammatory, antimicrobial, astringent, bitter, emmenagogue, expectorant, hepatic, laxative, oxytocic (stimulator of childbirth)

Indications: This is one of our most useful remedies; it owes much of its value to the tonic effects it has on the body's mucous membranes, making it a great help in all digestive problems, from peptic ulcers to colitis. Its bitter stimulation helps in loss of appetite. Goldenseal improves all catarrhal conditions, especially those of the sinuses. The alkaloids it contains stimulate bile production and secretion and give it antimicrobial properties. Berberine, an alkaloid found in goldenseal and a number of other herbs, has antibiotic, antispasmodic, carminative, cholerectic, immunostimulatory, hypotensive, sedative, and uterotonic activity. *Hydrastis canadensis* has traditionally been used during labor to help contractions; this means that it should be avoided during pregnancy. Apply goldenseal externally to help conjunctivitis, earache, eczema, itching, and ringworm.

Combinations: In stomach conditions, goldenseal combines well with chamomile and meadowsweet. For uterine hemorrhage, it is best combined with beth root. Combine with witch hazel as an external wash for irritation and itching; combine with mullein for ear drops.

Preparations and Dosage: To make an infusion, pour 1 cup boiling water over ½–1 teaspoon of the powdered herb and steep for 10–15 minutes. Drink three times a day.

As a tincture, take 1 ml three times a day.

HOP *(Humulus lupulus)*

Part Used: Flowers (strobiles)

Actions: Antimicrobial, antispasmodic, astringent, hypnotic, sedative

Indications: Hop is a remedy that has a marked relaxing effect upon the central nervous system. It is used extensively for the treatment of insomnia. It eases tension and anxiety and can be used where tension leads to headache, restlessness, and possibly indigestion. As an astringent with these relaxing properties, it can be used in conditions such as mucous colitis. Avoid it, however, where there is a marked degree of depression. Use its antiseptic action externally for the treatment of skin ulcers.

Preparations and Dosage: To make an infusion, pour 1 cup boiling water over 1 teaspoon of the dried flowers and steep for 10–15 minutes. Drink one cup at night to induce sleep. Strengthen this dose if needed.

As a tincture, take 1–4 ml three times a day.

LADY'S MANTLE (Alchemilla mollis)

Parts Used: Leaves and flowering shoots

Actions: Anti-inflammatory, astringent, diuretic, emmenagogue, vulnerary

Indications: Widely used in folk medicine throughout Europe, Lady's mantle reduces pains associated with menstruation. It also eases the symptoms of menopause. As an emmenagogue, it stimulates proper menstrual flow; in the seemingly paradoxical way of many herbal remedies, Lady's mantle is also a useful uterine astringent, used in both menorrhagia (excessive menstrual blood loss) and metrorrhagia (uterine hemorrhage). Its astringency is used to treat diarrhea, as well. Lady's mantle makes a good mouthwash for sores and ulcers and a gargle for laryngitis.

Preparations and Dosage: To make an infusion, pour 1 cup boiling water over 2 teaspoons of the dried herb and steep for 10–15 minutes. Drink one cup three times a day.

To make a stronger remedy for diarrhea or as a mouthwash or lotion, boil the herb for a few minutes to extract all the tannin. Strain, and drink one cup three times a day.

As a tincture, take 1–2 ml three times a day.

LEMON BALM (Melissa officinalis)

Parts Used: Dried aerial parts (or fresh when in season)

Actions: Antidepressive, antimicrobial, antispasmodic, carminative, diaphoretic, hepatic, nervine

Indications: Lemon balm is an excellent carminative herb that relieves spasms in the digestive tract and is used in flatulent dyspepsia. Because of its mild antidepressive properties, it is primarily indicated where there is dyspepsia associated with anxiety or depression. The volatile oil appears to act on the interface between the digestive tract and the nervous system. Some herbalists describe the oil as being restorative to the nervous system, similar to oats. Use lemon balm in migraine headaches that are associated with anxiety-induced palpitations, insomnia, neuralgia, and tension.

Lemon balm has a tonic effect on the heart and circulatory system, causing mild vasodilation of the peripheral vessels and lowering blood pressure. Use it in feverish conditions such as influenza. Hot water extracts of the herb have antibacterial and antiviral properties; use a lotion-based extract for skin lesions due to herpes simplex.

The hormone-regulating effects of lemon balm are well documented in the laboratory. Freeze-dried aqueous extracts inhibit many of the effects of thyroid stimulating hormone (TSH) on the thyroid gland by interfering with the binding of TSH to plasma membranes and by inhibiting the enzyme iodothyronine deiodinase. It also inhibits the receptor-binding and biological activity of immunoglobulins in the blood of patients with Graves' disease, a condition that results in hyperthyroidism. It will not, however, induce hypothyroidism in people with normal thyroid function.

Preparations and Dosage: To make an infusion, pour 1 cup boiling water over 2–3 teaspoons of the dried herb or 4–6 fresh leaves and steep, covered, for 10–15 minutes. Take one cup in the morning and one in the evening, or when needed.

As a tincture, take 2–6 ml three times a day.

MARSH MALLOW (Althaea officinalis)

Parts Used: Root and leaf
Actions: Anti-inflammatory, demulcent, diuretic, emollient (skin softener), expectorant

Indications: An abundance of mucilage makes marsh mallow an excellent demulcent. The roots traditionally have been used mainly for the digestive system, while the leaves are used more for the urinary system and lungs. It helps in all inflammatory conditions of the gastrointestinal tract, including colitis, gastritis, inflammations of the mouth, and peptic ulceration. Use marsh mallow leaves to help relieve cystitis, urethritis (inflammation of the urethra), and urinary gravel (small, gravel-like kidney stones), as well as bronchitis, irritating coughs, and respiratory catarrh. Use the herb externally in drawing ointments for abscesses and boils or as an emollient for varicose veins and ulcers.

Preparations and Dosage: To make an infusion, place 1–2 teaspoons of the root in 1 cup cold water and steep overnight. Drink as needed to alleviate the discomfort of heartburn.

As a tincture, take 1–4 ml three times a day.

MEADOWSWEET *(Filipendula ulmaria)*

Parts Used: Aerial parts

Actions: Antacid, antiemetic, anti-inflammatory, antirheumatic, astringent, carminative

Indications: Meadowsweet is one of the best digestive remedies available and is used in a holistic context to treat many conditions. It protects and soothes the mucous membranes of the digestive tract, reducing excess acidity and easing nausea. It is used in the treatment of gastritis, heartburn, hyperacidity, and peptic ulceration. Its gentle astringency is useful in treating diarrhea in children. The presence of aspirinlike chemicals explains meadowsweet's action in reducing fever and relieving the pain of rheumatism in muscles and joints.

Combinations: Combined with chamomile and marsh mallow, meadowsweet is very soothing for a whole range of digestive problems. For musculoskeletal conditions, consider combining with black cohosh, celery seed, and willow bark.

Preparations and Dosage: To make an infusion, pour 1 cup boiling water over 1–2 teaspoons of the dried herb and steep for 10–15 minutes. Drink one cup three times a day or as needed.

As a tincture, take 1–4 ml three times a day.

MILK THISTLE *(Silybum marianum)*

Part Used: Seeds

Actions: Cholagogue, demulcent, galactogogue, hepatic

Indications: Milk thistle can increase the secretion and flow of bile from the liver and gallbladder. Research showing that the herb contains constituents that protect liver cells from chemical damage has supported its traditional use as a liver tonic. Milk thistle is used in a range of liver and gallbladder conditions, including hepatitis and cirrhosis, and may have value in the treatment of chronic uterine problems. A wealth of research done in Germany is revealing exciting data about milk thistle's role in the reversal of toxic liver damage as well as protection from potential hepatotoxic agents. As its name implies, milk thistle promotes milk secretion and is perfectly safe for breastfeeding mothers.

Preparations and Dosage: To make an infusion, pour 1 cup boiling water over 1 teaspoon of the ground seeds and steep for 10–15 minutes. Drink one cup three times a day.

As a tincture, take 1–2 ml three times a day.

A POWERFUL PROTECTOR

A number of chemical components of milk thistle have a protective effect on liver cells. All are flavones and flavo-lignins; the best studied of these is silymarin. Silymarin has been shown to lessen and sometimes reverse the effects of highly toxic alkaloids, such as phalloidine and amanitin from the death cap mushroom *(Amanita phalloides)*. Silymarin's pharmacodynamics, site, and mechanism of action are becoming well understood, providing insights into the metabolic basis of this herb's activity, an activity long known and used by medical herbalists.

Oak Bark *(Quercus alba)*

Part Used: Bark
Actions: Anti-inflammatory, antiseptic, astringent
Indications: Use oak bark wherever a strong astringent is indicated — for example, in unresponsive diarrhea or dysentery. With its high tannin content it might be too strong in some situations, however, causing constipation. Use oak bark as a gargle for laryngitis, pharyngitis, and tonsillitis. Use it as an enema to treat hemorrhoids and as a douche for leukorrhea. Oak bark's primary indication is acute diarrhea, for which it is taken in frequent small doses.
Preparations and Dosage: To make a decoction, add 1 teaspoon of the bark to 1 cup of cold water and bring to a boil. Simmer gently for 10–15 minutes. Strain, and drink one cup three times a day.

As a tincture, take 1–2 ml three times a day.

Peppermint *(Mentha x piperita)*

Parts Used: Aerial parts
Actions: Analgesic, antiemetic, anti-inflammatory, antimicrobial, antispasmodic, aromatic, carminative, diaphoretic, nervine
Indications: Peppermint is an excellent carminative, has a relaxing effect on the muscles of the digestive system, combats flatulence, and stimulates bile and digestive juice flow. Use it to relieve flatulent dyspepsia, intestinal colic, and associated conditions. The volatile oil acts as a mild anesthetic to the stomach wall, which allays feelings of nausea. It helps to relieve the nausea and vomiting of both pregnancy and travel sickness. Peppermint can play a role in the treatment of ulcerative conditions of the bowels. It is a traditional treatment of colds, fevers, and influenza and is often used as an inhalant for the temporary relief of nasal catarrh. Peppermint might help headaches associated with digestion. As a nervine, it eases anxiety and tension. In dysmenorrhea, it relieves the pain and eases associated tension. Use peppermint externally to relieve itching and inflammations.

Preparations and Dosage: To make an infusion, pour 1 cup boiling water over 1 heaping teaspoon of the dried herb and steep for 10 minutes. Drink as often as desired for any of the above conditions.

As a tincture, take 1–2 ml three times a day.

RHUBARB ROOT *(Rheum palmatum, R. palmatum* var. *tanguticum)*

Part Used: Rhizome
Actions: Astringent, bitter, laxative
Indications: This is not the common garden rhubarb. Rhubarb root has a purgative action for use in the treatment of constipation; it also has an astringent effect following the primary action. Therefore, it has a truly cleansing action upon the gut, removing debris and then toning and providing antiseptic properties. *Note:* Rhubarb root might impart a red or yellow color to the urine. Do not use during pregnancy unless instructed by a qualified herbalist.
Preparations and Dosage: To make a decoction, add ½–1 teaspoon of the root to 1 cup cold water and bring to a boil. Simmer gently for 10 minutes. Strain, and drink one cup morning and evening.

As a tincture, take 1–2 ml three times a day.

SENNA *(Senna alexandrina)*

Parts Used: Leaves and dried fruit pods
Actions: Stimulating laxative
Indications: Senna is a powerful cathartic used in the treatment of constipation. It works through a stimulation of intestinal peristalsis. Remember that the cause of the constipation must be diagnosed and treated and not simply temporarily relieved with senna.
Preparations and Dosage: To make an infusion, steep the dried pods or leaves in warm water for 6–12 hours. Two different species are sold commercially; if using Alexandrian senna pods, use 3 to 6 pods in 1 cup of water; if using Tinnevelly senna, use 4 to 12 pods in 1 cup of water.

As a tincture, take 2–4 ml before bedtime.

SLIPPERY ELM *(Ulmus rubra)*

Part Used: Inner bark
Actions: Anti-inflammatory, astringent, demulcent, emollient, nutrient
Indications: Slippery elm bark is a soothing, nutritive demulcent that is perfectly suited to sensitive or inflamed mucous membrane linings in the digestive system. Use it to treat colitis, enteritis, gastric or duodenal ulcer, gastritis, and similar conditions. It is often used as a food during convalescence, as it is gentle and easily assimilated. When used for diarrhea, slippery elm will soothe and astringe at the same time. Externally, this herb makes an excellent poultice for abscesses, boils, or skin ulcers.
Preparation and Dosage: To make a decoction, combine 1 part of the powdered bark with 8 parts water, mixing the powder in a little of the water initially to ensure it will mix. Bring to a boil and simmer gently for 10–15 minutes. Drink ½ cup three times a day.

VALERIAN *(Valeriana officinalis)*

Parts used: Rhizome, stolons, and roots
Actions: Antispasmodic, carminative, emmenagogue, hypnotic, hypotensive, nervine
Indications: This herb has a wide range of specific uses, but its main indications are for anxiety, nervous sleeplessness, and the bodily symptoms of tension such as muscle cramping or indigestion. It can be used safely in situations where tension and anxiety are causing problems. For some people valerian is an effective mild pain reliever.

Valerian enhances the body's natural slumber process. It also helps enhance rest times of wakefulness. Current research is confirming what herbalists have known for years: Valerian is one of the best sleep-improving remedies available.

Much of the research on valerian has centered on its relaxant effects upon smooth muscle. Because of this ability, it can be safely used to treat intestinal colic, muscle cramping, and uterine cramps. Valerian decreases both spontaneous and caffeine-stimulated muscular activity, and significantly reduces aggressiveness of animals.

Valerian is used worldwide as a relaxing remedy in hypertension and stress-related heart problems. There is an effect here beyond simple nerve relaxation, as it contains alkaloids that are mild hypotensives. The World Health Organization recognizes such uses.

Combinations: Italian researchers compared the relaxing properties of valerian and a number of other plants on the muscles of the digestive tract. Hawthorn and valerian had the greatest effects, followed by chamomile and passionflower. And a combination of all of these herbs acted in a synergistic way, being relaxing at low dosage levels.

VALERIAN AND SLEEP

The true nature of sleep remains a mystery. Everybody goes through stages of REM (rapid eye movement) where dreaming is associated with minor involuntary muscle jerks and eye movements, indicating that active processes are occurring in the brain. It is important not to suppress dreaming during this stage; the mind processes emotional experiences in those dreams, and the unconscious and conscious parts of the brain come into balance. While sleeping pills have a marked impact on REM, valerian is not powerful enough to suppress these necessary REM phases. Sleep assisted by valerian is more restful and rejuvenating.

Preparations and Dosage: To be effective, valerian has to be used in sufficiently high dosage. The tincture is the most widely used preparation; take 2.5–5 ml (½–1 teaspoon) 20 minutes before retiring. Increase to 10 ml if necessary. For situations of extreme stress where a sedative or muscle relaxant effect is needed quickly, take 1 teaspoon two or three times total at short intervals.

To make a hot infusion, pour 1 cup boiling water over 2 teaspoons of the dried herb. To make a cold infusion, pour 1 cup cold water over 2 teaspoons valerian root; steep for 8–10 hours. Using this method you can prepare the nighttime dose in the morning and prepare the morning dose at bedtime.

VERVAIN *(Verbena officinalis)*

Parts Used: Aerial parts
Actions: Antispasmodic, diaphoretic, galactogogue, hepatic, hypotensive, nervine tonic, sedative
Indications: Vervain strengthens the nervous system while relaxing tension and stress. It can ease depression and melancholia, especially when they follow an illness such as influenza. Vervain can treat seizures and hysteria. Use the herb as a diaphoretic in the early stages of fevers and as a hepatic remedy to help reduce inflammation of the gallbladder and jaundice. Use vervain as a mouthwash against tooth decay and gum disease. Do not use vervain during pregnancy.
Preparations and Dosage: To make an infusion, pour 1 cup boiling water over 1–3 teaspoons of the dried herb and steep for 10–15 minutes. Drink one cup three times a day.

As a tincture, take 2–4 ml three times a day.

WAX MYRTLE *(Myrica cerifera)*

Part Used: Bark of root
Actions: Astringent, circulatory stimulant, diaphoretic
Indications: Sometimes called barberry, this herb is a valuable astringent in diarrhea and colitis. It is also a good gargle for sore throats. As a douche it helps stop leukorrhea (a white or yellowish vaginal discharge). It has been used in the treatment of colds, flus, and other acute feverish conditions. Do not use this herb during pregnancy.

Preparations and Dosage: To make a decoction, add 1 teaspoon of the bark to 1 cup cold water and bring to a boil. Remove from heat and steep for 10–15 minutes. Drink one cup three times a day.

As a tincture, take 1–2 ml three times a day.

WILD LETTUCE *(Lactuca virosa)*

Part Used: Dried leaves

Actions: Anodyne, antispasmodic, hypnotic, nervine

Indications: The latex (white gel-like substance within the stems) of wild lettuce was at one time sold as "Lettuce Opium," quite an appropriate name! It is a valuable remedy for insomnia, restlessness and excitability (especially in children), and other manifestations of an overactive nervous system. As an antispasmodic it can be used as part of a holistic treatment for whooping cough and dry, irritated coughs in general. Wild lettuce relieves colic pains in the intestines and uterus, making it useful for dysmennorhea. Wild lettuce eases muscular pains related to rheumatism. It has also been used as an anaphrodisiac.

Combinations: For irritable coughs, combine with wild cherry bark. For insomnia, combine with valerian and pasqueflower *(Anemone pulsatilla)*.

Preparations and Dosage: To make an infusion, pour 1 cup boiling water over 1–2 teaspoons of the leaves and steep for 10–15 minutes. Drink one cup three times a day.

As a tincture, take 1–2 ml three times a day.

WILD YAM *(Dioscorea villosa)*

Part Used: Dried rhizome

Actions: Anti-inflammatory, antirheumatic, antispasmodic, cholagogue, diaphoretic, hepatic

Indications: At one time this valuable herb was the sole source of chemicals used as the raw materials for contraceptive hormone manufacture. In herbal medicine wild yam is a remedy that can relieve intestinal colic, soothe diverticulitis, and ease dysmenorrhea and ovarian and uterine pains. It is very useful in the treatment of rheumatoid arthritis, especially the acute phase in which there is intense inflammation.

Preparations and Dosage: To make a decoction, add 1–2 teaspoons of the herb to 1 cup cold water and bring to a boil. Simmer gently for 10–15 minutes. Drink one cup three times a day.

As a tincture, take 2–4 ml three times a day.

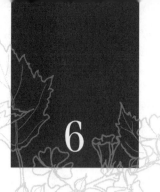

6

MAKING
HERBAL MEDICINES

There is nothing mysterious or even particularly clever about making healing formulations from plants. The pharmaceutical elite would have us think that to be of any use a medicine must be made by a Ph.D. wearing a white lab coat and then packaged with half an acre of rain forest material. Not so! If you can make a cup of tea and cook a meal that your friends would be willing to eat you are qualified. (If this is not the case, or if you've lost friends due to your lack of cooking skills, then perhaps the best place to start is with a book by Julia Child!)

The first way our ancestors used herbs was no doubt by eating the fresh plant. Over the thousands of years that humans have used herbs since then, we have developed other methods of preparing these plants. With our modern knowledge of pharmacology, we can make educated choices as to which of these processes to use to release the biochemical constituents that are all-important to healing — without insulting the integrity of the plant by isolating fractions of the whole.

Since healing takes place from within, the most effective way of using herbs is to take them internally. There are numerous ways to prepare internal remedies, but whether you're making a tea, a tincture, or a dry herb preparation, it is essential to work carefully to ensure you end up with what you want.

There are a couple of distinct advantages to making your own herbal medicines. First, you will get a sense of empowerment from being intimately involved in your own healing process. Second, the cost of homemade preparations is many times less than that of commercial medicines.

TEAS

There are two types of herbal teas, or water-based extracts of herbs: infusions and decoctions. There are some basic rules for choosing which method to use with what herb, but, of course, there are many exceptions.

Infusions are the method of choice for non-woody material such as flowers, leaves, and some stems, where the active ingredients are readily accessible. The denser the plant or individual cell walls, the more energy is needed to extract cell contents into the tea; therefore, the more heat-intense process of decocting is used for herbs that contain hard or woody material such as bark, nuts, or roots.

As with anything in the real world, not every herb falls neatly into one of these categories. This is especially true of roots that are rich in volatile oil, such as valerian root. The woodiness of the root suggests decocting, but if the roots are simmered the therapeutically important volatile oil would boil off. Therefore, an infusion is the preparation of choice for valerian root. As you can see, you must learn about the herb you intend to use in order to make the most appropriate preparation.

How to Make an Infusion

If you know how to make tea, you know how to make an infusion. Infusions are best for non-woody parts of the plant such as leaves, flowers, or green stems. If you're making an infusion of bark, root, resin, or seeds, it is best to powder them first to break down some of the cell walls, making them more accessible to water. If you're working with seeds, such as aniseed and fennel, bruise them slightly with a mortar and pestle before infusing to release the volatile oils from the cells. Infuse any aromatic herb, such as chamomile and peppermint, in a well-sealed pot to ensure that only a minimum of the volatile oil is lost through evaporation.

An infusion is the simplest method of utilizing both fresh and dried herbs. Fresh herbs have more water content than dried; when working with fresh herbs, substitute three parts fresh for one part dried. For instance, if the recipe calls for 1 teaspoon of dried herb, substitute 3 teaspoons of fresh herb.

To make an infusion:

Step 1. Warm a china or glass teapot by swishing hot water through it. Place about 1 teaspoon of the dried herb for each cup of tea into the warmed pot.

THE BEST HERBS FOR INFUSIONS

Herbal infusions make an exquisite addition to our lifestyles and can open a whole world of subtle delights and pleasures. They are not only medicines or "alternatives" to coffee, but can be delicious beverages in their own right. Everyone will have his or her favorite herbs; here are some of my favorites. Use them individually or in combination. Choose herbs based on both taste and medicinal properties.

Flowers: chamomile, elder flower, hibiscus, linden blossom, red clover
Leaves: lemon balm, lemon verbena, peppermint, rosemary, spearmint
Berries: hawthorn, rose hips
Seeds: aniseed, caraway, celery seed, dill, fennel
Roots: licorice

Step 2. Pour in 1 cup of boiling water for each teaspoon of herb and cover with the lid. Steep for 10 to 15 minutes.

It's usually best to drink medicinal herbal teas hot, but you can drink infusions cold as well. Make a cold infusion if you are working with mucilage-rich herbs, such as marsh mallow, which are sensitive to heat. For a cold infusion, the proportion of herb to water is the same, but let the infusion steep for 6 to 12 hours in a well-sealed pot of cool water. When a hot or cold infusion is ready, strain, and sweeten to taste if desired with a bit of honey, brown sugar, or a pinch of a pleasant-tasting herb such as licorice or stevia.

If you prefer not to deal with the messiness of loose leaves, make your own teabags by filling little muslin bags with herbal mixtures (take care to remember how many teaspoons of herb you put into each bag). As with ordinary teabags, pour boiling water over the bag and allow the herbs to steep for 10 to 15 minutes.

Make larger quantities of infusion in the proportion of 1 ounce of herb to 1 pint of water. Whenever possible, infusions should be prepared fresh, but if you do have any leftovers store them in glass containers in the refrigerator. The shelf life of infusions is not very long; any microorganism that enters the infusion will multiply and thrive in it. If you see any sign of fermentation or spoilage, discard the infusion. These telltale signs can vary, depending on the materials used. Generally, look for color or odor changes, clouding, condensation, and molding; all of these changes indicate spoilage.

How to Make a Decoction

If you select hard, woody herbs, making a decoction will ensure that the soluble contents of the herbs actually reach the water. To ensure that the constituents are transferred to the water, you will need more heat for the decoction process than for infusions.

To make a decoction:

Step 1. In a glass, ceramic, earthenware, or enameled metal pot or saucepan, place 1 teaspoon of dried herb for each cup of water. (For larger quantities, use 1 ounce of dried herb for each pint of water.)

Step 2. Add 1 cup of water for each teaspoon of dried herb. Bring to a boil and then simmer for 10 to 15 minutes or for the amount of time specified for the particular herb or mixture. If the herb contains volatile oils, cover the pot.

Step 3. Strain the herbs from the tea while still hot, sweeten if desired, and drink.

If you're preparing a mixture that contains both soft and woody herbs, prepare separate infusions and decoctions to ensure that the more sensitive herbs are treated accordingly. Combine the two liquids and drink.

TINCTURES

Extracts of herbs in alcohol or glycerin are called tinctures. Tinctures are much stronger, volume for volume, than infusions or decoctions, so the dosage is usually much smaller. Tinctures also have a longer shelf life, extract all of the soluble material from the plant, and tend to be less expensive than other preparations. Tinctures have the benefit of concentration, making them more convenient to take.

Tinctures are used in a variety of ways. You can take one straight or mix it with a cup of cool or hot water. When added to hot water, the alcohol in the tincture will largely evaporate, leaving most of the extract in the water. You can also add a few drops of tincture to a bath or footbath, use it in a compress, mix it with oil and fat to make an ointment, or use it to make suppositories and lozenges.

WINE-BASED TINCTURES

Another way to make a kind of alcohol tincture is to infuse herbs in wine. Even though these wine-based preparations do not have the shelf life of other tinctures and are not as concentrated, they can be both pleasant to take and effective.

How to Make a Tincture

Alcohol is a better solvent than water for most plant constituents; alcohol dissolves nearly all of the ingredients and acts as a preservative. Tinctures based on glycerin have the advantage of being milder on the digestive tract and are a good bet for people who would rather not ingest alcohol. However, glycerin does not dissolve resinous or oily materials well. As a solvent, glycerin is generally better than water but not as good as alcohol.

The method outlined here is a basic approach. Remember, if you are using fresh rather than dried herbs, use three times the amount. To make a tincture:

Step 1. In a glass container that can be closed tightly, place 4 ounces of finely chopped or ground dried herb. Pour 1 pint of 80-proof vodka over the herbs and cover tightly. If using glycerin as the solvent, make a mixture of ½ pint glycerin and ½ pint water (for fresh herbs, use a mixture of 75 percent glycerin to 25 percent water); pour this mixture over the herbs and cover the container tightly.

Step 2. Keep the container in a warm but dark place for at least two weeks and shake it once a day.

Step 3. Strain the liquid through a muslin cloth suspended in a bowl. Wring out all the liquid from the herbs. (The spent herbs make excellent compost!)

Step 4. Pour the tincture into a dark glass bottle. Close the bottle tightly and label with all ingredients and the date. Stored properly out of direct sunlight, the tincture will last many years.

DRY HERB PREPARATIONS

There a number of advantages to taking herbs in a dry form, mainly because you can avoid the taste of the herb while consuming the whole herb (including the woody material). Unfortunately, there are also a number of drawbacks:

- Dry herbs are unprocessed, and so the constituents are not always readily available for easy absorption. Unlike an infusion, during which heat and water help to break down the walls of the plant cells and dissolve the constituents, the digestive process of the stomach and small intestines is not guaranteed to break down plant cell walls.
- When the herb's constituents are already dissolved in liquid form, they are available a lot more quickly and begin their action sooner.
- Avoiding the taste of the herb can also be considered a drawback. For instance, bitter herbs work best when tasted, since their effects result from a neurological reflex. When bitters are put into a capsule or a pill, their action can be diminished or even lost.

Taking all these considerations into account, there are a number of ways to use herbs in dry form. Always be sure the herbs are powdered as finely as possible. Grinding guarantees that the cell walls are largely broken down and helps in the digestion and absorption of the herb.

The most convenient way to grind herbs is with a coffee or spice grinder; don't use the same one for your coffee or spices, as it can retain the scent and flavor of the herbs. Mortars and pestles are traditional options and look more attractive, but they sometimes require hard work to use. For larger quantities of herbs, a food processor is ideal.

Capsules

Gelatin capsules are a convenient way use powdered herbs. The capsule size depends on the amount of herbs prescribed per dose, the density of the plant, and the volume of the material. A size 00 capsule, for instance, holds about ⅙ ounce of finely powdered herb.

Filling a capsule is easy:

Step 1. Place the powdered herbs on a flat dish and separate the halves of the capsule.

Step 2. Move the halves of the capsules through the powder, scooping the herb into the two halves.

Step 3. Push the halves of the capsule together.

Capsules should be stored in a sealed container in a cool, dry place out of direct sunlight. This type of medicine is usually best taken with food, but the specifics will vary from herb to herb.

Pills

There are a number of ways to make pills, from the very simple to the complex. The simplest way to take an unpleasant remedy is to place the powder on a slice of fresh bread. Roll into a small ball shape. This method works most effectively with herbs such as goldenseal or cayenne.

BIBLIOGRAPHY

Brown, Donald. *Herbal Prescriptions for Better Health.* Rocklin, CA: Prima Publishing, 1996.

Ellingwood, Finley. *American Materia Medica, Therapeutics, and Pharmacognosy,* 1898. Portland, OR: reprinted by Eclectic Medical Publications, 1983

Hobbs, Christopher. *Foundations of Health: The Liver and Digestion Herbal.* Capitola, CA: Botanica Press, 1992.

Hoffmann, David. *The Complete Illustrated Holistic Herbal.* Shaftesbury, England: Element, 1996.

———. *An Elder's Herbal.* Rochester, VT: Healing Arts Press, 1992.

———. *The Herbal Handbook.* Rochester, VT: Inner Traditions, 1988.

———. *Successful Stress Control.* Rochester, VT: Healing Arts Press, 1986.

Keville, K. *Herbs for Health and Healing.* Emmaus, PA: Rodale Press, 1996.

Murray, Michael and Joseph Pizzorno. *Encyclopedia of Natural Medicine.* Rocklin, CA: Prima Publishing, 1990.

Soule, Deb. *The Roots of Healing: A Woman's Book of Herbs.* New York: Citadel Press, 1995.

Weiss, Rudolf. *Herbal Medicine.* Portland, OR: Medicina Biological, 1988.

RESOURCES

**National Digestive Diseases
Information Clearinghouse**
2 Information Way
Bethesda, MD 20892-3570
(301) 654-3810
Web site: www.niddk.nih.gov/
health/digest/digest.htm
*The National Digestive Diseases
Information Clearinghouse (NDDIC)
is part of the National Institutes of
Health under the U.S. Department of
Health and Human Services. The
clearinghouse provides information
about digestive diseases to people with
digestive disorders and to their fami-
lies, health care professionals, and the
public. NDDIC answers inquiries and
develops, reviews, and distributes
publications.*

American Liver Foundation (ALF)
75 Maiden Lane, Suite 603
New York, NY 10038-4810
(800) 465-4837
Web site: www.liverfoundation.org

**Crohn's & Colitis Foundation
of America, Inc.**
386 Park Avenue South,
17th Floor
New York, NY 10016-8804
(800) 932-2423 or
(212) 685-3440
Fax: (212) 779-4098
Web site: www.ccfa.org
E-mail: info@ccfi.org

**International Foundation for
Functional Gastrointestinal
Disorders (IFFGD)**
P.O. Box 17864
Milwaukee, WI 53217
(414) 964-1799 or
(888) 964-2001
Web site: www.iffgd.org
E-mail: iffgd@iffgd.org

INDEX

Page numbers in *italics* indicate illustrations; page numbers in **boldface** indicate charts.

OTHER BOOKS IN THE STOREY
MEDICINAL HERB GUIDE SERIES